For Thomas, who never flinched,
and for Hedda, his teacher

For my dear Anna —
who supports me
in red + green —

I love you + appreciate
you endlessly.

Chris
xxoo

Contents

Illustrations

Foreword

Chris Bobel's account of third-wave menstrual activism is a generational eye-opener. For a second-wave feminist like me, whose early goal in life was to have a full-time career and a family at the same time, menstruation was something to be minimized, managed, and made invisible. The idea of flaunting its bodily manifestations and making it the basis of political activism would have been unbelievable and retrograde to me. My generation gratefully seized on tampons and "the Pill" to accomplish the goal of making menstruation and birth control less of a bother. We soon learned to manipulate oral contraceptives so the bleeding days occurred at our convenience; I expect that I would have embraced the means of medically suppressing menstrual periods entirely had the drug Lybrel been available then. It was therefore with a bit of skepticism and a show-me attitude that I came to Chris Bobel's work on flaunt-and-fight menstrual activism.

Menstrual activists, Bobel notes, straddle several strands of feminism. Like radical feminists and body spiritualists, menstrual activists want to experience their bodies fully and naturally, and as eco-feminists, they also boycott, or "girlcott," commercial single-use products for reusable cups and homemade cotton pads. More significantly for feminist theory and practice, they directly and deliberately address conflicts among feminists. As Bobel says, "The menstrual activist struggle taps directly into the ongoing tug-of-war between feminists who embrace sexual difference theory and those who embrace gender theory." Some movement activists want to make menstruation everyone's issue, not just menstruators'. They want to include among the menstruators intersex people and transmen who bleed but do not identify themselves as women. By splitting femaleness and womanhood from menstruation, one branch of menstrual activism spills over into queer theory and challenges the standard sex/gender

binaries as limiting human expression and perpetuating gender inequality. In
the sense that disrupting these binaries is a core aspect of third-wave feminism,
these menstrual activists are an example of transformative feminist theory and
practice.

Third-wave feminism is, however, more than queer theory. Indeed, it is what
young contemporary feminists *do*. According to Bobel, third-wave feminist
practice demonstrates inclusion of all types of feminism, recognizes each
person's multiple identities and the consequent ambiguities and contradictions
in standpoints, and embraces living feminism in everyday activities, down to the
minutiae of choosing what method or product to use during menses. That is,
menstrual activism exemplifies third-wave feminism because it includes "'feminist spiritualists,' menstrual activists who work to reclaim menstruation as a
healthy, sacred, empowering, and even pleasurable experience for women," and
"radical menstruation" rebels who rail against the mainstream commercial
products most menstruators use.

While many second-wave feminists are uncomfortable with the gynocentric
orientation of feminist spiritualists, arguing that it is essentialist, many are also
uncomfortable with gender queering, contending that it makes women invisible
all over again. I see gender queering as potentially revolutionary. In *Breaking the
Bowls: Degendering and Feminist Change*, I advocate de-legalizing gender as a
basic social identifier and not sorting everyone into the conventional sex/gender
binaries, since that process sustains gender inequality.

When it comes to menstrual activism's eco-feminism, however, I am not
persuaded by the movement to do away with commercial products. Perhaps
I can't detach from my second-wave idea of making menstruation as convenient
as possible, but I can't see twenty-first-century women in developed countries
sewing their own menstrual pads and washing and reusing them. To me, and
I suspect to many who will read Bobel's book, that's throwing menstruators
back to the drudgery of pre-twentieth-century chores. It may be environmentalist and punk; it may be anticorporate and antiglobalization, but I wonder how
many ecofeminists and punk rockers are using menstrual keeper cups or pinning
homemade cloth pads into their panties. Maybe they agree that they *should* opt
for alternatives, but do they?

So, is menstrual activism a good example of third-wave feminism or is it
simply an exotic submovement—well intentioned yet fundamentally impracti-
cal? It seems to be both. It is environmentalist, anticorporate, anti–global capitalist, body oriented, and gender queer. It is rooted in everyday practices rather
than movement politics. But it is also an exotic submovement for all the same
reasons. The girlie culture so prevalent in third-wave feminism, with its
unapologetic use of cosmetics, high heels, and sexy clothes, is surely body oriented, but hardly environmentalist, anticonsumerist, or particularly gender

queer. And while it is true that third-wave feminism is inclusive enough to make room for menstrual activism, this little-known movement has a lot of work to do before it becomes a formidable impetus for social change.

Demographically, menstrual activism leaves out major groups of third-wave feminists—women of color and working-class women, in particular. Bobel found little attention to menstruation in Black feminism and other feminisms of color; she did find some interest in "holistic womb health" and Mexican and Native American folk medicine around menstruation, though not immediately and only in small numbers. For women of color and working-class women, as Bobel points out, making menstruation unobtrusive would be more in line with a striving for upward mobility than its celebration, although a concern for healthier products might be appealing.

Bobel's account of menstrual activists is a story of third-wave feminism and its conflicts and contradictions, especially around gender versus woman. She asks, "What should feminist activists do about the category 'woman'?" This is not a new question, of course, but she provides us with a new way of thinking about the answer. In her view, the place to see how menstrual activism furthers third-wave feminist practice and theory is in "radical menstruation's project of queering menstruation [as] a cutting edge activist approach to embodiment." That is, "woman" is deessentialized but bodies are valorized. Radically, these bodies are neither necessarily female nor necessarily woman identified. This attempt to reconcile gender queering and menstruation is quite paradoxical, but what remains to be seen is the reach of the movement. Certainly, someone who doesn't menstruate could care about the safety and environmental compatibility of femcare products, but do they have a place in a do-it-yourself campaign? Are males or postmenopausal women or male-to-female people going to make or wash cotton menstrual pads? Indeed, Bobel found little Internet interest by the trans community in issues of menstruation, leading her to wonder, "Perhaps the movement wants them, but do they want the movement?"

Bobel's book is not only about a little-known movement. It is also, as she points out, more provocatively a book about feminism in flux. So, in the end, what is the significance of menstrual activism to feminism? The feminist spiritualists join embodiment theory and practice in embracing women's menstruating bodies as beautiful and powerful. The radical genderqueers join feminist postmodernism in challenging the conventional binaries. Using "menstruators" in the narrower sense of people whose bodies bleed periodically rather than equating menstruation with womanhood goes along with the project of detaching sex (body, physiology) from gender (social identity and social status). The anticonsumerists and environmentalists in menstrual activism strengthen likeminded feminists active in other issue-oriented movements—animal rights, veganism, and antiglobalization, for example. Menstrual activism is thus very much part of the feminist third wave—inclusive, conflicted, and contradictory. Bobel's comprehensive account of the movement is thus an excellent entrée into understanding how contemporary feminists *do* feminism.

Judith Lorber, Professor Emerita
Graduate Center and Brooklyn College,
City University of New York,
Brooklyn

Acknowledgments

The paradox of crediting everyone while taking sole responsibility for the outcome is never more acute than for a researcher and writer. I must begin by acknowledging that there would be no book if already too-busy activists had not offered their time to a complete stranger. I am stunned by the generosity and good humor of more than seventy activists, from Kutztown, Pennsylvania, to Stockholm, Sweden. Many of these amazing people not only shared their lives but also swung the gate wide open so I could connect with others. Special thanks go to Yonah EtShalom, Kate Zaidan, Andrea Mickus (all of the Student Environmental Action Coalition [SEAC]), ALisa Starkweather, Chella Quint, adee, Miranda Resnick, Rina from Macalester, Anna Yang of the Red Web Foundation, Sissy Sparkle, Kami McBride, Breeze Harper, Emily Biting, Erin Wilkins, Karolina Bång, Miki Walsh, Brackin "Firecracker" Camp, Kristin Garvin, and Giovanna Chesler for going *way* above and beyond.

I warmly thank Madeleine Shaw of Lunapads, who volunteered to organize a contest to find the cover image. And because of Madeleine, I was privileged to consider the work of many talented and inspired artists who offered up their innovative work as possibilities. Ultimately, Helena González Sáez's image spoke to me most and I feel privileged that it graces the cover.

Jane Bobel of Jane Bobel Graphic Design (and not so incidentally, my big sister) is entirely responsible for the preparation of all interior images. Through this process, she endured an endless flow of my confused and conflicted e-mails. I, no doubt, abused any implicit familial contract of support.

Natalie Wysong served as a nurturing midwife to this manuscript's first full draft; Dori Gilbert and Perri Weinberg-Schenker both arrived right before this "baby" was born, smoothing out the citations and endnotes. And finally, Bobbe Needham—consummate and patient copyeditor—sent her out into the world.

My writing group, populated by the savviest group of feminist intellectuals this side of anywhere, deserves my deepest thanks: Sarah Sobieraj (who held my shaking hand more than once), Frinde Maher (who helped me see Platform 9 3/4) Anna Sandoval Girón, Susan Ostrander, Julie Nelson (who conjured the book's title), Jyoti Puri, and JoAnne Preston.

Hedda Hartl came all the way from Germany on multiple occasions to feed our family, wash our clothes, and care for our baby so I could work. Without her selfless nurturance offered up quietly and steadily, I'd still be merely writing a book proposal. "I miss you" is an understatement.

While all my students school me regularly, my research assistants deserve special mention. Coral Waters, Ginn Norris, Jenna McGlynn, Natalia Cooper, Jessie Baird (look for her in chapter 7), Bonnie Gerepka, and Sarah Okolita each poked into the dark holes in the conceptual framework and helped me produce a fuller, richer, and more complex argument. Sarah's intrepid archival sleuthing in particular was fundamental to chapter 3.

I thank my mentor and guardian angel Jean Humez whose inspired pencil helped me produce clearer focus and punchier critique. Meredith Evans's expertise regarding third-wave feminism sharpened my own thinking; chapter 1 is largely indebted to her. My appreciation goes to Thomas Hartl, who extracted the data on the contemporary FemCare industry. I also thank my colleagues at UMass Boston who make that *other* part of my professional life—teaching and service—endlessly meaningful and pleasurable.

Andrea Scarpino, Kevin Allred, Gayle Sulik, Doreen Drury, Ann Blum, and Jan Thomas said yes when I asked, and their handprints are all over the good parts. Liz Kissling's careful reading of the first full draft triggered the growth spurt I needed at a crucial crossroads. My early writing group, comprised of Marianne McPherson, Katrina Zippel, Katja Guenther, Sheryl Medlinger, Rachel Powers, and Katie Fraser, were there when menstrual activism was little more than white noise. Phyllis Mansfield and Peggy Stubbs gave me substantive feedback and publishing venues that pushed my work out there and bolstered my confidence to ask better and clearer questions.

Through the wonders of Skype, I leaned on Jessica Fields, Sarah Sobeiraj, and Tina Fetner—scholars who pull back the curtain on productivity and demonstrate that writing needn't be tortured but admit that it often is.

Members of Sociologists for Women in Society and of the Society for Menstrual Cycle too numerous to name protected me from the chill of scholarly isolation (hard to find a research area more fraught with stigma than *feminist* studies of *menstruation*). I can't thank you enough. In particular, Verta Taylor's mentoring found me when I was lost in the conceptual woods, and Judith Lorber's supportive comments about my early work validated the project and served as a touchstone when my confidence flagged. I am truly honored to have Judith's foreword introduce the book.

I must acknowledge the College of Liberal Arts Dean's Grant Fund and the UMass Boston Healey Grant Program, as well as the Women's Studies Research Center (WSRC) at Brandies University, for their support of this work, including Shula Reinharz and members of the Science and Gender work group, especially kindred souls and whip-smart scholars Bridgette Sheridan and Christine Cooper (the brilliant feedback of the latter pulled me back from the edge of a cliff, manuscript in hand).

I couldn't live with myself if I didn't thank: my pals, John Sanbonmatsu, Suzanne Cox, Julie Duhigg, and Judy Ingalls, and again, Andrea Scarpino, who kept me as close to sane as anyone can be when on the tenure track; Cheryl Moloney, transcriptionist extraordinaire; and Sandy Crooms, who believed in the project and graciously led me to the Rutgers University Press door when an earlier publisher restructured. And, finally, I thank Doreen Valentine, who immediately "got" the project and made it possible for you, dear reader, to find this book in your hands (or on your screen).

Finally, my girls near, Gracie and Zoe, and my boy far, Craig, are the inspiration for my seeking (if not yet finding) work-life balance. My partner, Thomas Hartl, never called me a hypocrite when I bitterly complained about my own period while writing this book, and that's representative of the kind of steadfast and bottomless support he offers me when I am researching, writing, and doing everything else that matters.

———

A much-abridged version of chapter 3 was published as "From Convenience to Hazard: A Short History of the Emergence of the Menstrual Activism Movement, 1971–1992," *Health Care for Women International* 29, no. 7 (2008): 738–754. A very early portion of chapter 5 was published as "'Our Revolution Has Style': Menstrual Product Activists 'Doing Feminism' in the Third Wave," *Sex Roles: A Journal of Research* 54, nos. 4/5 (2006): 331–345. And a fragment of the same appeared as "Resistance with a Wink: Young Women, Feminism, and the (Radical) Menstruating Body," in *Gendered Bodies: Feminist Perspectives from Birth to Death*, ed. Judith.Lorber and Lisa Jean Moore (Los Angeles: Roxbury Publishing, 2006), 87–91.

New Blood

Introduction

MICHIGAN WOMYN'S MUSIC FESTIVAL, 2001

On a Thursday morning in August, I am thumbing through the impressive list of workshops offered at the Michigan Womyn's Music Festival, highlighting those that grab me. I discover one titled "Ax Tampax," which promises to "explor[e] the politics, issues, and experiences of menstruation including discussion of the dangers of disposable products and the presentation of safer alternatives."

The politics of menstruation? Dangers of products? Alternatives? What?

I'm intrigued and circle "Ax Tampax" with my pink highlighter. Two days later, I join about two-dozen women who listen with rapt attention to the twenty-something workshop presenter. Representing "the Bloodsisters: a radical wimmin's health project from Montreal," a woman who goes by the name adee is dressed in a beige slip trimmed in lace, a straw cowboy hat, and a pair of cowboy boots.[1] With tremendous ease and clarity, she plunges into the myriad risks associated with conventional FemCare: dioxin poisoning, microlacerations, yeast infections, endometriosis, toxic shock syndrome, and the prolific waste produced by both the production and the disposal of single-use products.[2] adee accuses the FemCare industry of sexism. They don't care about women's health and safety, she says. Then she plays show-and-tell with a dizzying array of alternative menstrual products—sponges, cups, and assorted cloth pads in leopard print and tiger stripe.

Who knew?

I stroke the flannel of the handmade reusable pad and take in the scene. I listen to various tales of transformation: "I'll never use tampons again! I love my Keeper!" one woman exclaims.[3] My mind slips back to something I read recently: "People wonder who is carrying on the legacy of the women's movement and they look to the same old haunts to find the answers. The problem is, they are looking in the wrong places."[4] Perhaps, I couldn't help thinking, we should be looking *here*. Might not the women's movement be carried on in places like this workshop, by activists like adee?

On Saturday, the last night of the festival, during the infamous parade that snakes through the festival grounds, my jaw drops as the self-titled Red Brigade moves past me. A group of women—about twenty strong in various states of undress (typical for the festival)—are decorated with red paint and red police tape marked "DANGER." The Blood Brigade is noisy and powerful, and their demonstration meets with hoots and hollers of approval from the crowd. I am transfixed by this feisty group—their red, their rage, their guts to take on a cultural taboo with such, well, flair. They are sassy; they have style. About half the participants hoist signs made of cardboard and painted with red paint. The slogans include "Tampax Evil!" "Join the Red Revolution," "We Have Our Own Wings," and "Get Corporations Out of Our Cunts." I appreciate the signs' creativity and bold use of language, but my eyes fix on a less inflammatory but highly poignant message: "The Personal Is Political." It is, of course, familiar to me, this famous slogan first penned by Carol Hanisch in the heady early days of the second wave of the U.S. women's movement. But in this context, "The Personal Is Political" takes on a new meaning, connecting the past, the present, and, perhaps, the future of the women's movement. I wonder if I am witnessing what's called "third-wave feminism." Is this a continuation of second-wave feminism, forged in the late 1960s and 1970s? Or is there something different about the way these activists interpret and enact their feminism? As a professor of women's studies, I was familiar with a wide range of feminist activism, such as the antiwar work of Code Pink, the medical practice interventions of the Intersex Society of North America, and the Lesbian Gay Bisexual and Trans Rights (LGBT) lobbying of the Human Rights Campaign. But where does activism like the Bloodsisters' fit? What, exactly, does doing feminism look like in the twenty-first century, and what does it portend about the future of the women's movement?

Compelled by these questions, I decided to look more closely at the Bloodsisters and the menstrual activism movement of which they are a part. This research, a quest for clarity and reconciliation, set me on a journey to study up close and in depth the kind of feminism embodied by those sassy Bloodsisters and their "The Personal Is Political" poster—an image that, for me, symbolizes a contemporary movement at once groundbreaking and rooted in the recent past. Like Jo Reger, a sociologist who studies the contemporary women's movement, I follow second-waver Gloria Steinem, who quipped, "If you want to know about young feminists, you should ask one."[5] Four years of fieldwork, hours of archival research and textual analysis, and sixty-five in-depth interviews later, I still may have more questions than answers. But what has become clear is this: Menstrual activism is not only an interesting (if little-known) movement in its own right, but it also offers insight into the U.S. women's movement today, especially third-wave feminism. What many call third-wave feminism, the contested next

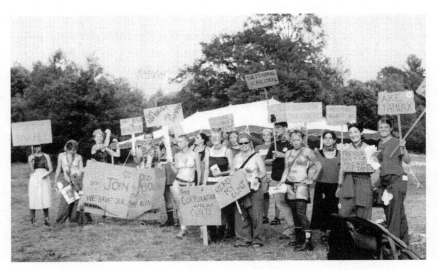

Figure 1. The Red Brigade, Michigan Womyn's Music Festival, Hart, Michigan, 2001. Photo by the author.

stage in the U.S. women's movement populated by mostly (though not exclusively) young women and men, demonstrates an interesting blend of tactical continuity and ideological innovation.[6] While most of the actions I observed in the menstrual activism movement had second-wave precedents (though their targets often differed), these third-wavers broke ground most notably in the ways they troubled the relationships between key categories of identity.

PALPABLE TENSIONS AMONG FEMINISTS

The lively and contentious debate regarding third-wave feminism is a minefield. Forged in the 1990s, third-wave feminism is arguably the newest expression of feminist thought and practice. Even though most third-wave writing has taken the form of personal narrative, common questions have emerged to form a critical body of scholarship.[7] What is third-wave feminism, really? Is it a set of values distinct from second-wave feminist theory, a genuine ideological departure, which in turn requires practical innovation? Or is third-wave feminism simply a generational shift, little more than a linguistic convention that marks two distinct historical moments within one movement? These questions are simultaneously fundamental and complex, and a lot is at stake in how we go about answering them.

Even the term "third wave" is contested as an apt description of the newest phase in the U.S. women's movement, given the conflict among feminists who cannot agree if there is indeed such a thing as a "third wave" of feminism. In response some, like Jo Reger, choose to refer to "contemporary feminism." But

I prefer the language "third wave" for two reasons. First, I find "contemporary" merely a code for "third wave" that avoids the contentious debates occurring now within and between feminisms. Second, the term "contemporary" is misleading; contemporary feminists include Gloria Steinem and Eve Ensler, but I would not characterize either as "third-wavers." Thus, I willingly step into the fray by using the albeit imperfect and fraught terminology "third-wave feminism."[8]

Those who identify as third wave endeavor to distinguish themselves from the feminist pack. To quote Vivian Labaton and Dawn Lundy Martin, editors of an anthology of third-wave writing titled *The Fire This Time: Young Activists and the New Feminism*: "Young feminists have shed the media-espoused propaganda about feminists but have taken to heart the criticism from women of color that the second-wave was not racially or sexually inclusive enough. The addition of third-wave in front of the term feminism for them is reclamation—a way to be feminist with a notable difference."[9] In her examination of the generational conflict between the waves, Astrid Henry found that some third-wavers describe second-wavers as "puritanical, dated, dowdy, [and] asexual."[10] Many third-wavers see the feminist movement as stalled, in desperate need of new energy and much richer racial, ethnic, and sexual diversity. In a low-budget documentary on radical cheerleading (a popular third-wave feminist street protest tactic) made by a group of young feminists, second-wave activism is dismally described as "too often just a bunch of exhausted, bored, but well-intentioned people standing and holding signs while some angry white man ordered them around with a bullhorn."[11] The common refrain that follows such depictions is "something's got to change." A new breed of feminism, young feminists assert, is necessary to address the deficiencies of a second-wave feminism that has passed its prime. Third-wavers believe they present a new face of feminism, a feminist expression necessarily more inclusive, more active, more popularly accessible, and thus better equipped to mobilize resources—both ideological and tactical—against "postfeminist" backlash.

In response, some feminists, including those who identify as second wave and those who sit uneasily between the waves (such as scholars Astrid Henry, Catherine Orr, and Lisa Maria Hogeland), point out the impoverishment of third-wave renderings of the women's movement, a tragic ahistoricism that, they claim, dooms progress (not to mention offends a lot of feminist activists). Some second-wave feminists shake their heads and wring their hands about the future of feminism. These young feminists, they groan, are letting slip the gains already made. For example, Natalie Fixmer and Julia Wood admonish third-wavers for practicing what Jennifer Baumgardner and Amy Richards call "everyday feminism" while neglecting legal issues, issues at the heart of much second-wave activism.[12] In a *Time* magazine feature on the demise of feminism, Gina Bellafante captured what she called the "Old Guard feminist" dismay with newer feminist expressions: It's not surprising that Old Guard feminists, surveying their legacy, are dismayed by what they see. "All the sex stuff is stupid," said Betty Friedan. "The real problems have to do with women's lives and how you put together work and family."[13] Susan Brownmiller, author of *Against Our Will*, a book that pioneered the idea that rape is a crime of power, counterpoints with: "These are not movement people. I don't know whom they're speaking for. They seem to be making individual bids for stardom."[14]

Feminism has heard this complaint before—the sense that members of a generation have failed to adequately acknowledge the strides made by those in the previous era. In 1910, U.S. suffragist Anna Howard groused: "It is everywhere the same question—the young people come into the work with the greatest lack of respect for the older people; they think we have made great blunders all these years and have kept the work back; that now they are going ahead in their sweet and beautiful way."[15]

When we step back and survey these debates, it becomes clear that second-wavers and third-wavers are both engaging in the same sort of generalizing. Representatives from one wave tend to overlook the diversity within the other, while they minimize (or ignore) what the other wave has achieved. Points of connection between the waves are neglected, as is the work of feminists who do not fall easily into either the second- or third-wave categories. Troubled by those left out of the talk of waves, Kimberley Springer asks whether we can even conceive of waves of the movement without erasing the work of women, especially women of color, who work between the waves.[16]

Sociologist Nancy Naples joins Springer in her critique of the limits of the wave metaphor. Naples studied women from diverse racial-ethnic, class, and cultural backgrounds whose organizing expanded notions of political work beyond conventional forms of social protest. Many of these struggles, she notes, "are now significant aspects of third-wave feminist activism." To avoid obscuring such contributions and, consequently, "offer[ing] a narrow conceptualization of what counts as feminism," she advocates differentiating between waves of protest and what Nancy Whittier calls "political generations," a concept that acknowledges that while activists may come from the same era, there are variations within that era demarcated by their entry points (roughly divided into regular intervals).[17] Yet another critique of the wave discourse is articulated by Lisa Jervis, founding editor of a popular third-wave periodical, *Bitch: Feminist Response to Pop Culture*: "What was at first a handy dandy way to refer to feminism's history, present and future potential with a single metaphor has become shorthand that invites intellectual laziness, an escape hatch from the hard work of distinguishing between core beliefs and a cultural moment."[18] Speaking in terms of waves simultaneously creates and hardens arbitrary divisions while it elides authentic differences. After all, writes Devoney Looser: "If there is now a growing body of writing on second-wave and third-wave feminist experiences, beliefs, and platforms, little has been written on the traffic between each so-called camp."[19]

Astrid Henry took up this challenge when she interrogated the "matrophor" used in much third-wave feminist writing. She found that the mother-daughter trope, which positions second-wave feminists as mothers and third-wavers as daughters, produces a generational distinction that is rigid, monolithic, and oppositional. Furthermore, such distinctions are hierarchical and essentialist. They lock mothers and daughters in power struggles over who speaks for embodied feminism, reify the maternal-feminine link, and exclude feminist men.[20] I agree, and I join with Henry in a project of "troubling" the too-easy, too-tidy divide between feminists. Rather than try to settle the debate, I seek to better understand the tensions that shape the conflicts among feminists. Furthermore, my position as an in-betweener enables me to bring a distinctive lens to this project, seeing value (and limitation) in both waves, and to help inch us toward common feminist ground.

New Blood: Third-Wave Feminism and the Politics of Menstruation is an empirical study. Although analyses of the third wave have begun to accumulate, few studies rely on in-depth observation of third-wave feminism in action. Thus, I chose a primarily ethnographic study of a particular movement within the movement, which, as it unfolded, shed light on tensions the extant scholarship has identified between the emerging third and the established second wave. But let me be clear. This is not a study that seeks to resolve the tensions or end the debates. In fact, I am not convinced that the debates about the waves are productive. Might they be another red herring, an intramovement struggle that distracts from the real work of feminism—to end gender oppression? With this study, I seek rather to understand the consequences of a set of tensions within feminism that just won't go away.

Controversial and understudied, menstrual activists like the Bloodsisters allege the hazards of commercial FemCare to both women's bodies and the environment and promote alternatives that are less costly and more healthful for users and the planet. Fundamentally, they rail against the dominant cultural narrative of menstruation that constructs a normal body process particular to females as disgusting, annoying, taboo, and best kept out of sight and out of mind. Their work, I show, has historical precedents in the second wave. To best access the world of the menstrual activists, I embarked on a multidisciplinary, multimethod study that both troubles the very notion of waves in the women's movement and points to the ways in which younger feminists today are a force to be reckoned with. Other analysts of the women's movement have identified continuities between U.S. feminism's waves.[21] My aim here is to flesh out such analyses by looking closely at an example of feminism on the ground. Through this examination, I not only identify endurance and transformation in contemporary feminist activism, but I also capture their consequences, an aspect lacking in the existing literature.

A SOLUTION IN SEARCH OF A PROBLEM?

As I grew to know the menstrual activists, I found that in spite of their complex, provocative, controversial, and colorful character, they had escaped scholarly attention. While the topic of menstruation has generated some interest in the social sciences and humanities, especially the examination of cultural attitudes about the menstrual cycle and rhetorical analyses of media representations of menstruation and related products, to date no one has devoted a study to the diverse range of strategic efforts young women and girls use to challenge the culture of menstruation, including how they care for their menstruating bodies and the ideological inspiration at the root of these efforts.[22] Thus, study of menstrual activism yields important insights into the evolution of social movements and feminist epistemology, a system of knowledges in constant flux. In addition, because menstrual activism is a body-centered movement, studying it connects with the exploding interdisciplinary scholarship on the body, particularly women's bodies, and the origin and persistence of sex and gender differences.[23]

Menstrual activism rejects the construction of menstruation as a problem in need of a solution, or as historian Joan Brumberg puts it, little more than "a hygienic crisis."[24] Typically, a young woman's first period is marked not with celebration, but with a quick, furtive talk about supplies (read: pads, tampons, and maybe Midol). Acceptable menstrual discourse (if that phrase is not oxymoronic) is limited to complaints about cramps, jokes about mood swings, and, increasingly, the appeal of continuous oral contraception to suppress menstruation. With FDA approval of Seasonale in 2003 and the more recent approval of Lybrel during spring 2007, the menstrual cycle has become an especially hot topic.[25] On April 20, 2007, the *New York Times* ran a front-page article titled "Pill That Eliminates the Period Gets Mixed Reviews." The article stimulated a wave of media attention, including blog entries, a CBS news segment, a position statement issued by the Society for Menstrual Cycle Research, and an angry article in the magazine *Reason* that accused feminist critics of menstrual suppression of being elitists who wish to deny women an option they desire. What is rarely addressed in the media coverage, however, are these profound questions: Why, exactly, do nearly all women hate their periods more than their other bodily processes? How do culture, gender ideology, and consumerism shape these reactions?

As I demonstrate in chapter 2, these questions are at the core of menstrual activism and drive activist efforts to confront negative representations of menstruation, which impede the development of safe products, the distribution of comprehensive information, and honest, informed dialogue about this bodily process. The activists have their work cut out for them, given that many women aren't interested in claiming the menstrual cycle but are eager to banish it. For example, a 2003 study found that one-third of women surveyed indicated that they would eliminate their periods permanently if they could.[26] When I ask my female students what aspect of womanhood they like least, they quickly volunteer: "Having a period!" Contrary to these views, menstrual activists assert that menstruation is a healthy bodily process—a vital sign—that should not be cursed, masked, or suppressed. For some, it can even be enjoyed and used as a tool to develop what is called "body literacy." At the very least, they argue, what journalist Karen Houppert calls "the culture of concealment" surrounding menstruation must be penetrated.[27] How else can we mobilize to demand safer, more environmentally friendly products? How else can consumers challenge the big pharmaceutical companies' incursion into the menstrual cycle, marketing an increasing number of drugs that manipulate the body merely for convenience's sake? If we can't *talk* about menstruation, how can we possibly make productive noise about menstrual culture and its interventions?

A Little-Known Movement That Echoes the Past

There *has* been noise about menstrual culture for longer than many of us may realize. Menstrual activism is an outgrowth of mid-to-late twentieth-century feminist women's health activism. The women's health movement resists the androcentric, so-called objectivity of the medical establishment and fights to provide women with alternatives in their health care.[28] Over time, the movement built upon this foundation and expanded its critique, attracting more constituencies, among them consumer rights advocates also skeptical of the burgeoning FemCare industry's lack of commitment to menstruator safety. Early movement activity was pioneered by feminist-spiritualists who worked at the level of individual self-transformation, framing menstruation as a source of untapped female power and woman-centered identification. Calling for a conceptual shift, they made art and created ritual, music, and poetry. And, I discovered, they are still at it today—one of the two active wings of the contemporary menstrual activism movement.[29]

Reform-minded feminist health activists began to question menstrual product safety in the late 1970s. They were galvanized to join with consumer rights advocates in the wake of the 1980 toxic shock syndrome (TSS) outbreak, with 813 cases of menstrual-related TSS linked to tampon use, resulting in thirty-eight deaths.[30] By 1983 more than 2,200 cases had been reported to the CDC.[31] While some activists faced off with industry and government officials in the interest of tampon safety, other activists entered the movement bringing new priorities and approaches. The environmentalists among them attacked the FemCare industry as an egregious polluter and admonished menstruators to seek more sustainable alternatives, such as all-cotton, unbleached tampons and pads. In the 1990s, the radical menstruation wing of the movement sprouted. Aligned with third-wave feminism and a punk youth ethos of alienation, radical menstruation activists resist what they see as corporate control of menstruation and promote the use of reusable menstrual products (extremists, called "free bleeders," use nothing at all).

While the reformist tactics of women's health and consumer rights activists have become a part of history, today's menstrual activism employs a rich variety of tactics, from the sacred to the ribald and the practical to the abstract. The movement's two wings: the feminist-spiritualists, who have endured since the 1970s (gathering new recruits through the years), and what I am calling the radical menstruation activists. This submovement illuminates current tensions in the women's movement. My focus is primarily on the radical menstruation activists who shift from working with the industry to produce safer products—as earlier activists did when they donned their suits and flew to Washington, D.C., to confront the FDA and FemCare industry representatives—to turning *away* from the industry and deploying art and performance laced with humor to raise awareness and challenge the dominant paradigm. For activists affiliated with this wing, refusing to play along with the menstrual status quo and talking directly to menstruators, not to industry, is revolutionary. While earlier activists attempted to reform the FemCare industry and feminist-spiritualists focus on self-transformation, radical menstruation activists promote the radicalization of both thought and protest action. For example, at the University of North Carolina–Chapel Hill, campus-based radical menstruation activists staged a Tampon Send Back campaign outside the student union and distributed literature titled "What Your Mother Never Told You about Tampons." In St. Paul, Minnesota, approximately forty students at a small liberal arts college hand-sewed reusable cloth menstrual pads while debunking the bizarre and common myths of menstruation. On the campus of Colorado State University, a ragtag group of radical cheerleaders, donning pink netting and feather boas, performed a series of cheers that expose the hazards of conventional FemCare and promoted the use of alternative options.[32]

At Once Old and New

Ax Tampax
In spirit of challenging and collapsing
The insidious nature of the corporate monster
That gobbles and trashes and fucks us over . . .
In response to the dirty business . . .
We have made this recipe book.
As an act of resistance to the system
That tramples over the homegrown d.i.y. style
We are sick of how they co-opt our life
To spit out into franchises . . .
To over package our needs into taxed luxuries . . .
We are sick of the garbarators
That insists to dismember . . .

We are sick of how it insists to hide
And disguise our experiences
Fuck the mark up they make on their lies . . .
Down with the inventors of necessities!
To the uprising when we stop popping tampons
And the popping big business medicines . . .
We fuck the poisons
That kill our free remedies . . .
When we fuck the complacency
To build the uprising . . .
To bleed and use weeds
To stop feeding the corporate greed
When we ax tampax and what it embodies.[33]

This piece penned by adee and titled "Ax Tampax Poem Feministo"—part poetry, part manifesto, and part statement of conscience—shouts from the pages of a zine titled *Red Alert #3* that the Bloodsisters Project produced and disseminated in 2002. The zine makes an ideal forum for disparaging what some activists call "the corporate creeps." Menstrual activists use zines to educate readers about alternatives, usually through a favorite third-wave tactic, first-person narrative, as in, "Let me tell you about the first time I used a Keeper." And while third-wave activists can claim zines as a relatively recent activist mouthpiece, the use of independent publishing in the feminist movement has a long, rich history. Early women's liberation tracts, such as the *Redstockings Manifesto*, were self-published and distributed similarly. Other tactical continuities across the waves abound. DIY (do-it-yourself) menstrual care, such as making your own menstrual pads, is reminiscent of the tradition of self-help gynecological care pioneered by feminist health activists of the second-wave. (Picture a roomful of women receiving hands-on instruction on how to properly examine one's own cervix.) Humor and performance also characterize tactics endemic to both the second wave and the third. When we see such continuities, writes Nancy Naples, we complicate "the firm differentiation between the waves of movement activism that has dominated recent feminist discourse."[34]

Tactical continuity is not the only mark of interwave unity. Always a feature of the U.S. women's movement, the white dominance persistent across its waves appears in the menstrual activism movement as well. Indeed, one of the most salient critiques advanced by emerging third-wave feminism has been U.S. feminism's historic inability to produce a racially, ethnically, and culturally diverse movement.[35] Nearly all the menstrual activists I observed and 91 percent of those I interviewed identified as white. How can we make sense of menstrual activism's whiteness? What does it suggest about the persistence of a particular raced dynamic in the U.S. women's movement—a dynamic with deep roots and a painful history? In an exploration of the development of race segregation in the U.S. women's movement, Wini Breines argues that white women's racism (in spite of explicit denunciations of racist thought and action), the rise of the Black Power movement, and the development of identity politics all factored into the divide between white and black movement participants.[36] Women of color were similarly marginalized, finding the singular focus on women's oppression a privilege limited to white women.[37] Are today's feminists shackled to this legacy?

The absence of women of color, at least on the surface of the movement activity I encountered, is certainly a feature of the menstrual activism movement. At the same time, a disproportionate number of queer-identified activists, most, but not all of whom are white, populate the movement. How to explain these numbers? Here, I draw on and expand Evelyn Higginbotham's notion of "sexual respectability"—a standard imposed on and internalized by black women in their bid for respect in the context of racist society.[38] This standard is not limited to black women, I venture, but applies to all women of color to some degree. Such a standard public linkage of the body with taboo is too risky. At the same time, queer activists aligned with LGBT movements inhabit a site where challenges to socially acceptable expressions of sexuality are breached. For some queer menstrual activists, inhabiting the social and discursive location of outsider forms a politics of transgression central to movement activity. This, of course, poses special challenges for queer menstrual activists of color. Thus, violations of norms in the sphere of sexuality, I suggest, support rather than impede the risk-taking and norm-breaking necessary to their engagement in menstrual activism.

The theme of interwave continuities, both tactical and demographic, is a key feature of menstrual activism. However, at the same time that particular links between the so-called waves emerge, there *is* something new and different about the way menstrual activists do feminism today—suggesting that a transformation in the women's movement is indeed afoot. Within the menstrual activist movement, there is a tension at work between the feminist-spiritualists and the radical menstruation activists that goes to the heart of the *politics* of the social construction of gender. This tension plays out in the different ways activists frame menstruation's definitional status. Some writer-activists affiliated with the feminist-spiritualists, like Erica Sodos, regard the menstrual cycle as a rite of passage for all women and a definitional experience, even a criterion, for womanhood. This framing of menstruation esssentializes women's bodies, assuming that menstruation is necessarily a feature of all women's experiences and thus a political and practical concern for every woman.

But not all women menstruate, and not only women menstruate. Post-menopausal women, women posthysterectomy, and some athletes, for example, do not menstruate, and some preoperative transmen do menstruate (as do many intersexuals). Recognizing these facts, a growing number of menstrual activists, especially those linked to punk and third-wave feminist communities, find the "I bleed, therefore I am a woman" discourse problematic. Inspired and informed by the rapidly burgeoning transgender, genderqueer, and intersex rights movements and by theoretical paradigms, such as feminist philosopher Judith Butler's idea of gender performativity popularized in the 1990s, they challenge essentialist constructions of womanhood in their work, carefully choosing their language and using their words to do what one campus activist called "gender education, you know, queering the binary."[39] For example, by referring to "menstruators" instead of "women," these activists "are making bleedin' everyone's issue" (per a popular activist slogan) by expanding menstruation beyond the confines of gender. This linguistic move expresses solidarity with women who do not menstruate, transgender men who do, and intersexual and genderqueer individuals. Refusing to equate menstruation with womanhood, such activists challenge the hegemony of the essentialized gender binary even in the context of what is generally taken to be a nearly universal embodied "women's issue." In this way, radical menstrual activism acts as a feminist project with the potential to undermine gender as a stable category. If even menstruation can be "queered," then the perceived necessity of the patriarchal two-gender system erodes. They "live Judith Butler" by translating theory into practice in the context of feminism on the ground.[40]

This strategy, provocative and bold, destabilizes the status quo, but can a movement rooted in a critique of the patriarchal construction of menstruation afford to erase the category "woman"? The menstrual activist struggle taps directly into the ongoing tug of war between feminists who embrace sexual difference theory and those who embrace gender theory. How do we, after all, conceptualize the end of women's oppression? If activism is necessarily informed by theory, this question cannot be ignored. Must the differences between women and men be articulated for feminist activism to exist, or should we throw out the very categories that construct these differences? Menstrual activism—populated by activists who subscribe to both sexual difference and gender theories—offers an on-the-ground illustration of what happens when theory becomes practice.

The feminist-spiritualists' work centers on celebrating what they see as the uniqueness of womanhood. Women will break free from oppression when they claim authority over their essential embodiment, they posit. In contrast, radical menstruation activists, consistent with third-wave aims of blurring boundaries, deploy a gender-neutral discourse of menstruation as they resist corporate control of bodies. For them, spiritualist-inspired self-transformation is inadequate. To achieve true liberation, "menstruators" must reject both essentialism *and* the commodification of the body.

Finally, the menstrual activism movement supplies a second illustration of troubling or "queering" boundaries as a third-wave feminist project. I agree with

U.S. women's movement scholar Nancy Whittier who, like me, recognized a large number of queer-identified people attached to third-wave feminism. Noting that sexual orientation is just one of the ways the movement is queer, she observed: "Criticism of identity politics was central to the third-wave and built directly in the anti-identity politics of the late 1980s and early 1990s. Although third-wave grassroots feminism is diverse in sexual identity, it is in many ways a 'queer' movement because of this approach to identity."[41] For Whittier, what is especially queer about what she calls "grassroots feminism" is not its sexual diversity (though that is important) but its refusal to claim labels or markers such as "feminist," "activist," and "progressive." What happens to our understanding of a movement when it refuses to be named?

Obviously, this is an exciting time in feminist history.

Menstrual activism helps us see what's at stake in the spirited debates about what to do about gender and the ongoing struggles to engage a truly racially, ethnically, and economically diverse movement of social change advocates around a common issue. While every feminist classroom and journal discusses exploding gender categories, the conversation lingers in the abstract. After more than thirty years of feminist debate, we aren't clear what this ideological position *looks* like when we actually *do* feminist activism. How can we talk about body-based discrimination, for example, without talking about women as women—even with all the differences within and among women? At the same time, how can we not afford to incorporate a questioning of fundamental categories like gender as we develop feminist agendas for the twenty-first century?

CHAPTER 1

Encountering Third-Wave Feminism

The Clarence Thomas–Anita Hill debacle of 1991 stirred the pot of feminist emotion. With rapt and often lascivious interest, the American public watched the televised Senate nomination hearings during which conservative African American nominee Clarence Thomas responded to accusations of sexual harassment. His accuser was a former colleague, African American Anita Hill, who alleged that on repeated occasions, Thomas made sexually charged comments and pursued her for dates, which she rebuffed. The sordid story, told and retold with crowd-pleasing detail, fired debates in countless kitchens, on shop floors, in break rooms, and in classrooms. For many feminists, some donning "I Believe Anita" t-shirts, the hearings revealed entrenched public ignorance and persistent myths about sexual harassment. But when Thomas characterized the hearings as a "high-tech lynching for uppity blacks who in any way design to think for themselves," many feminists, myself included, felt conflicted.[1] Was sexual harassment thrust into the national spotlight at the expense of a black man's ascendance to a high-profile government post? If so, was it impossible to confront sexism without participating in racism? Ultimately Hill's allegations were insufficient to block Thomas's confirmation, an outcome that left many feminists enraged. Among those angered was Rebecca Walker, daughter of legendary feminist writer and activist Alice Walker. In a 1992 *Ms.* magazine article, Walker crafted a feminist response to the notorious hearings in the form of an impassioned call to action. Urging young feminists to resist pronouncements that they inhabit a postfeminist era and to take up the mantle of feminist activism, she wrote: "Let Thomas' confirmation hearings serve to remind you, as it did me, that the fight is far from over. Let this dismissal of a woman's experience move you to anger. Turn that outrage into political power." She famously concluded her essay with the words: "I am not a post feminism feminist. I am the third-wave."[2] This is one story of the origin of the term "third-wave feminism."

But there are other accounts. Jo Reger, editor of *Different Wavelengths: Studies of the Contemporary Women's Movement*, notes that Walker is often credited with the term's origin but also points to sociologist Lynn Chancer's appeal a year earlier for a third wave of feminism to transcend the defensiveness of 1980s feminism.[3] Astrid Henry, author of *Not My Mother's Sister: Generational Conflict and Third-Wave Feminism*, locates a still earlier use of the term in a 1987 essay by Deborah Rosenfelt and Judith Stacey titled "Second Thoughts on the Second Wave." The article, published in the journal *Feminist Studies*, traced the myriad changes in feminism throughout the late 1970s and 1980s and observed that "the specific agendas of what some are calling a third wave of feminism are already taking shape."[4]

The conflicting stories of third-wave feminism's founding are emblematic of a deeper confusion about the meaning of "third wave." It is easier to locate what third wave is *not* than what it is. A centerpiece of third-wave discourse is the claim that third-wave theory and praxis are both markedly different from those of the second wave. For instance, Naomi Wolf, in her book *Fire with Fire: The New Female Power and How to Use It*, prods readers to shift from what she regards as the "victim feminism" of the second wave—a politics focused on women's disempowerment—to what she calls "power feminism." Wolf's brand of feminism deemphasizes oppression and instead focuses attention on women's expanding opportunities.[5] Another example of the third wave standing apart from feminism's second wave is evident on the home page of 3rd WWWAve: Feminism for the New Millennium, which states: "We are the 20- and 30-something women who have always known a world with feminism in it. We are putting a new face on feminism, taking it beyond the women's movement that our mothers participated in, bringing it back to the lives of real women who juggle jobs, kids, money, and personal freedom in a frenzied world."[6]

Leslie Heywood and Jennifer Drake, editors of the first scholarly collection on the third wave, titled *Third-Wave Agenda: Being Feminist, Doing Feminism*, also mark a difference in their attempt to theorize the emerging third wave when they focus on the ways that contemporary feminism operates as a project in decolonization and one that "changed the second wave of the women's movement for good."[7] The reference to decolonization is not solely about women claiming their agency, but also about feminism itself unlearning the racism, classism, and heterosexism that many third-wavers attribute to the second wave. Rightly crediting second-wave feminists of color such as Gloria Anzaldúa, bell hooks, Angela Davis, Barbara Smith, and Chela Sandoval, and others who exposed the second wave's lack of racial-ethnic diversity and inability to engage intersectional analyses that see race, class, and gender as interlocking systems of oppression, third-wavers call for a more inclusive movement that reckons fully with complexities of identity and experience. Still other third-wavers mark the third wave as distinctive in the way it locates the site of social change. Doubting the effectiveness of second-wave-style political action in the context of contemporary sociopolitical landscapes, many third-wavers find the realm of the personal more appealing and more promising as a site of radical transformation, and thus replace attempts at institutional change with attempts that address the context of culture and the realm of the everyday.

But who is the third wave? Who is initiating this break with feminism's recent past? This question, too, produces varied responses. For example, Jennifer Baumgardner and Amy Richards, authors of the feminist call-to-arms *Manifesta: Young Women, Feminism, and the New Future*, define the third wave as a movement populated by "women who were reared in the wake of the women's liberation movement of the seventies."[8] For Heywood and Drake, an even more precise (and limiting) definition of movement participants serves, capturing the generation of feminists born between 1963 and 1974.[9] Avoiding a demarcation based on age, but still marking generational differences, Rory Dicker and Alison Piepmeier, editors of *Catching a Wave: Reclaiming Feminism for the 21st Century*, assert that "the third-wave consists of those of us who have developed our sense of identity in a world shaped by technology, global capitalism, multiple models of sexuality, changing national demographics, [and] declining economic vitality."[10] Henry posits that the "'third-wave' has frequently been employed as a kind of shorthand for a generational difference among feminists, one based on chronological age," though she argues that the term more appropriately represents a "new" feminism that departs from the second wave, regardless of age.[11]

There are those, however, who resist such tidy distinctions and tend less toward chronological and more toward ideological and practical departures. Dicker and Piepmeier observe that, "typically, the third-wave is thought of as a younger generation's feminism, one that rejects traditional—or stereotypical—understandings of feminism and as such is antithetical or oppositional to its supposed predecessor, the second-wave." But in a gesture toward movement overlap, they characterize the third wave as "a movement that contains elements of second-wave critique of beauty culture, sexual abuse, and power structures while it also acknowledges and makes use of the pleasure, danger, and defining power of those structures."[12] This tension between past and present recurs in descriptions of third-wave feminism, a tension that is just beginning to produce what makes third wave distinctive. According to Judith Lorber:

> Third-wave feminism plays with sex, sexuality, and gender. In that sense, it is similar to postmodern feminism. It is inclusive of multiple cultures and men, and so continues multicultural/multiracial feminism and feminist studies of men. But it is rebellious when it comes to radical feminism. It rejects the sense of women as oppressed victims and heterosexual sex as dangerous. It does not valorize mothers or the womanly qualities of nurturance, empathy, and caretaking. Instead, third-wave feminism valorizes women's agency and female sexuality as forms of power.[13]

Lorber's analysis joins a small but growing number of scholarly analyses devoted to making sense of third-wave feminism. They include a special issue of *Hypatia* published in 1997; a cluster of articles in a 2004 issue of *National Women's Studies Association Journal*; Heywood and Drake's *Third-Wave Agenda*; Dicker and Piepmeier's *Catching a Wave*; Stacy Gillis, Gillian Howie, and Rebecca Munford's *Third-Wave Feminism: A Critical Exploration*, which the authors claim is "the first to bring the critical eye of the academy to bear upon third-wave feminism rather than it belonging to those who identify as 'third-wavers"; Amber Kinser's edited collection *Mothering in the Third-Wave*; Henry's *Not My Mother's Sister*; and a growing number of journal articles, including one by Kimberly Springer that ponders third-wave black feminism through an analysis of three texts by young black feminists written in the 1990s.[14] But "with some notable exceptions," as Reger has pointed out, "most of [the literature] focused on cultural analyses of contemporary feminism and less on empirical investigations of feminist communities."[15] Her sociologically informed edited collection *Different Wavelengths* and this book seek to fill that void.

Still, the hottest debates about what third-wave feminism is and is not are taking place in the context of collections of first-person narratives written by those who most identify with the newest expression of feminism. To relay a sense of the breadth of this literature, I list them in order of publication: *Bulletproof Diva: Tales of Race, Sex, and Hair* (1994), *To Be Real: Telling the Truth and Changing the Face of Feminism* (1995), *Listen Up! Voices from the Next Feminist Generation* (1995), the Australian *DIY Feminism* (1996), *Mama's Girl* (1998), *Body Outlaws: Young Women Write about Body Image and Identity* (1998), *Letters of Intent: Women Cross the Generations to Talk about Family, Work, Sex, Love, and the Future of Feminism* (1999), *When Chickenheads Come Home to Roost: My Life as a Hip-Hop Feminist* (1999), *Turbo Chicks: Talking Young Feminisms* (2001), *Colonize This! Young Women of Color on Today's Feminism* (2002), *We Don't Need Another Wave: Dispatches from the Next Feminist Generation* (2006), and *Third Wave Feminism and Television: Jane Puts It in a Box* (2007). The titles alone make very clear the third wave's investment in separating itself from the past—"today's feminism," "the next generation," "the new feminism," and the "new generation" all communicate that something new has arrived and it demands to be taken seriously.[16] But what is this something new? What, precisely, are the distinguishing features of this so-called new breed of feminism? To answer this question, Meredith Evans and I performed a thematic analysis of key third-wave texts we found representative of the range of the popular third-wave first-person genre. We elected to analyze the first collection to arrive on the scene, *To Be Real*; the first (and only) collection of third-wave narrative written exclusively by women of color, *Colonize This!*; the enduring *Listen Up!* (now in its second, expanded edition); and the activist-oriented and relative newcomer, *The Fire This Time*. It was our aim to uncover a more current definition of what

third-wave feminism means to the authors represented in third-wave antholo-
gies by searching for and interpreting the contributors' own definitions of
feminism. That is, we were invested in constructing a coherent definition of
third-wave feminism from the voices of those who identify most closely with it.
Our analysis produced four key themes that we found best captured the distinctive values, priorities, passions, and character of third-wave feminism as
expressed in this body of writing. They are inclusion, multiplicity, contradiction,
and everyday feminism.

Inclusion: Everyone under One Big Feminist Tent

Inclusion is a cornerstone of third-wave feminism. Indeed, third-wavers are
committed to "debunk[ing] the myth that there is one lifestyle or manifestation
of feminist empowerment" and to "defy[ing] stereotypes," while "creating a feminist movement that speaks to and represents the experiences of all women."[17]
This inclusive feminism seeks to redefine both feminism and gender roles to suit
women's lives rather than mold women to fit a particular feminist ideal.[18]
According to Pandora Leong, a contributor to *Colonize This!* the feminist "tent
holds scores of perspectives" and not only accepts but also celebrates all forms of
feminism.[19] Anna Bondoc, a contributor to *To Be Real*, describes her aim of want-
ing to "develop a politics of wholeness and three-dimensionality" so that she can
be in the "real world with the rest of the sinners and fools where we can get down
to some serious work." Bondoc explains that we have to be able to have faults
and still be able to claim feminism. In the down-to-earth prose characteristic of
third-wavers, she writes: "If the small-waisted, big-chested, white-capped tooth,
porcelain-skinned woman is the unattainable ideal of modeldom, then the
progressive ideal is equally unattainable: racist-free, classist-free, 100 percent
antihomophobic, angry and able to fully articulate every political issue."[20]

Inclusion suggests an absence of restrictions on how or when to be a feminist.
This is a feminism that does not judge or place boundaries on movement participants, thus moving away from dichotomies and political rigidity and allowing
for multiple possibilities. Inclusion is essential to building movement strength
and solidarity and appealing to would-be activists for whom the feminist label
felt too narrow and restrictive.

Of course, issues of inclusion have always been a concern of feminists. From
Sojourner Truth's "Ain't I a Woman?" speech at the 1851 Ohio Women's Rights
Convention, which exposed the double standards of femininity, to Rita Mae
Brown's 1969 statement describing the homophobia within the National
Organization for Women, feminists have been challenging the women's move-
ment to expand its borders.[21]

Perhaps the most impenetrable barrier to access to feminism is the privileg-
ing of so-called academic feminism. In an attempt to shape a stronger, more

inclusive movement, third-wavers reject the intellectual and professional elite that dominates much of feminist writing. For example in her fat-positive essay "It's a Big Fat Revolution," Nomy Lamm carves out a space for a raw, real discourse that breaks with what she calls "the universe of male intellect" ostensibly adapted by feminist academics: "If there's one thing that feminism has taught me, it's that the revolution is gonna be on my terms. The revolution will be incited through my voice, my words, not the words or the universe of male intellect that already exists. And I know that a hell of a lot of what I say is totally contradictory. My contradictions can coexist, cuz they exist inside of me, and I'm not going to simplify them so that they fit into the linear, analytical pattern that I know they're supposed to."[22] Although I challenge the conflation of "male" with "academic," which denies the tremendous amount of feminist scholarship by, for, and about women, as well as the plentiful numbers of public intellectuals and scholar-activists who refuse to distinguish their academic from their activist labors, I appreciate Lamm's point. Since the establishment of what is called the "intellectual arm of the women's movement"—women's and gender studies—academic feminism's bid for legitimacy has rendered much of the discourse inhospitable to all but the elite few. Feminism in some ways has become a specialized discourse. However, rejecting "the universe of male intellect" must not necessarily translate to anti-intellectualism. On this point, Catherine Orr accuses Lamm of "degrad[ing] anything that resembles intellectual labor," a criticism I've repeatedly heard leveled against third-wave feminists.[23] In fact, some of my colleagues choose not to teach third-wave literature in their classes because much of it takes the form of personal narrative. As one colleague complained to me, "How rigorous is a bunch of essays written by a bunch of young women gazing at their own navels?" While I will concede that there is some naval gazing and at times a dearth of analysis that adequately contextualizes individual experience, third-wave writing does express, in the aggregate, an earnest attempt to construct a feminist movement that all people can imagine themselves a part of. The writing expresses this value of inclusiveness through the use of personal stories expressed in candid, accessible, jargon-free language. This is a feminism that not only claims to be inclusive, but also demonstrates this value through its discursive practices.

MULTIPLICITY: BRINGING OUR WHOLE SELVES TO THE TABLE

A movement predicated on inclusion requires a reckoning with multiplicity that acknowledges human complexity. Without attention to multiplicity, after all, inclusion is impossible. This theme of understanding, examining, and accepting diverse experiences and standpoints surfaces as integral to the movement. Third-wavers embrace and celebrate their differences and acknowledge the multiple identities of each feminist or "fragmentation . . . as a place of power" through attention to the intersections of gender, race, class, and sexuality and all forms of oppression.[24] In this conceptualization, feminism is understood in the broadest terms and predicated on an understanding of the interconnectedness of oppressions and domination. In "Virtual Identity," a piece that explores the contemporary feminist politics of identity, Mocha Jean Herrup writes: "We realize that to fight AIDS we must fight homophobia, and to fight homophobia, we must fight racism, and so on."[25]

For third-wavers, there is no single feminist issue, but a constellation of interrelated issues that must be addressed simultaneously. As Audre Lorde observed: "There is no such thing as a single-issue struggle because we do not live single-issue lives." In the same vein, Labaton and Martin point out that "to demand that people focus on one area of concern without recognizing the interconnection of multiple issues would be to demand a level of self-abnegation that does not mirror the way these issues are experienced in our daily lives." As women, we must be able to "bring our whole selves to the table," declares Sonja Curry-Johnson, and to do that, it is essential to gain an understanding of the connection to underlying power structures. In another powerful essay that explores the complexity of identity politics, Danzy Senna explains how multiplicity is lived in her life: "I have come to understand that my multiplicity is inherent in my blackness, not opposed to it, and that none of my 'identities" are distinct from one another. To be a feminist is to be engaged actively in dismantling all oppressive relationships. To be black is to contain all colors. I can no longer allow these parts of myself to be compartmentalized, for when I do, I pass, and when I pass, I 'cease to exist.' "[26]

These writers insist that class, race, gender, and sexuality are not singular entities and cannot be separated within individuals; therefore, one should not expect that they can or should be separated in social justice work. They envision the "new" women's movement as accessible and relevant to everyone committed to ending oppression.

As even the casual observer of feminism could note, third-wave feminists cannot claim to have discovered intersectionality and the inescapable interconnectedness of issues. Feminists of color, working-class feminists, lesbian feminists, and others have long recognized the absolute necessity of what Patricia Hill Collins famously termed "the matrix of domination."[27] And while women who experience racism, classism, heterosexism, and other forms of oppression have always understood the impossibility of isolating gender-based discrimination from these, many white, middle-class, and straight women have been slow to make this connection; the women's movement thus became, for many, a white middle-class thing." Third-wave feminism outfaces the comfortable privilege that permits the luxury of working on what some call just women's issues, a forced separation premised on a myth that few women believe: that women's experiences are standardized. Third-wavers, particularly feminists of color, express frustration with a women's movement that fails to attract racially and ethnically diverse women. A feminism will inevitably fail that asks women to align with other women with whom they have less in common than they have with the men in their communities with whom they resist racism and ethnocentrism. As the Combahee Black Feminist Collective in a 1974 "Black Feminist Statement" asserted:

> Although we are feminists and lesbians, we feel solidarity with progressive black men and do not advocate the fractionalization that white women who are separatists demand. Our situation as black people necessitates that we have solidarity around the fact of race, which white women of course do not need to have with white men, unless it is their negative solidarity as racial oppressors. We struggle together with black men against racism, while we also struggle with black men about sexism.[28]

In this tradition, third-wave feminism works to foreground the intersections that shape experience, thus fully acknowledging how a truly progressive women's movement cannot separate gender from other dimensions of identity in the fight for social justice.

CONTRADICTION: AT ONCE COLONIZER AND COLONIZED

To embrace inclusion and multiplicity, one must be ready to reckon with the ensuing contradictions and potential conflicts among and within individuals in the movement. "Contradiction," inevitable in an inclusive and diverse movement, is arguably the most uttered word associated with third-wave feminism. Third-wavers want to accept and embrace the contradictions and ambiguities that exist within society and within themselves as individuals. Cristina Tzintzun captures this idea when she states in the lead essay of *Colonize This!*: "I am mixed. I am the colonizer and the colonized, the exploiter and the exploited. I am confused yet sure. I am a contradiction." Rebecca Walker, whose very name is fused with third-wave feminism, claims that by "facing and embracing their contradictions and complexities and creating something new and empowering from them," third-wave feminists move "away from dualism and divisiveness." This brings us closer to inclusion and multiplicity. Embracing contradiction means simultaneously acknowledging how we are, depending on our varying social contexts, oppressed and oppressive. In her contribution to *Listen Up!* Christine Doza explains it this way: "I need to know that every minute of every day I am being colonized, manipulated, and ignored, and that minute by minute I am doing this to others who are not shining white and middle class. There is a system of abuse here. I need to know what part I'm playing in it." Honoring differences and accepting the contradictions that exist are essential to maintaining inclusiveness and to avoiding the divisiveness that thwarts the building of a cohesive movement.[29]

As Nancy Naples points out: "Naming and navigating feminism's contradictions has become a primary theme of the third-wave." One of these contradictions is tied up in a fundamental—perhaps *the* fundamental—concept at the core of feminist theorizing: the category "woman." Gillis, Howie, and Munford note that the first- and second-wave fixation on woman as "both the object and subject of discourse" led feminists to question the very concept, because it "seemed too fragile to bear the weight of all contents and meanings ascribed to it." This questioning, they argue, caused a shift within the women's movement that led to even more foundational contestations about "the nature of identity, unity and collectivity," challenging what many third-wavers came to regard (albeit ignorantly) as the received truths of feminism, such as "a good feminist necessarily rejects men."[30] This questioning necessarily exposed the contradictions that shape day-to-day living, even (perhaps especially) for those who identify as feminists. Throwing off these contradictions as incompatible with feminism has been an aim of third-wave feminism; this shedding of the rules of consistency is part of a more general rejection of dogmas and dichotomies, real or imagined, attached to what third-wavers see as second-wave theory and practice.

For example, while third-wavers actively critique consumer culture, they defend (and even celebrate) their participation in it.[31] In her foreword to *Sisterhood, Interrupted: From Radical Women to Grrrls Gone Wild*, a playful romp through the history of the last thirty-plus years of the U.S. women's movement, Baumgardner unapologetically juxtaposes her activist work (addressing an audience of UCLA feminists) with her grooming rituals (conforming to dominant feminine beauty standards): "It's funny. Just before writing this foreword, I got an extreme bikini wax in Los Angeles with my writing partner and fellow feminist Amy Richards."[32] Here, in typical third-wave style, she confronts her readers with the possibility that feminists can at once play along with the rules of gender display and work aggressively for social justice. Provoking those who assume that participation in vain personal-care rituals is incompatible with feminism, she pushes back against a feminist dogma that she sees as counterproductive to building a diverse movement.

In my undergraduate course "Introduction to Women's Studies," I typically invite a panel of feminist-identified former students to share their thoughts about what feminism means to them. I do my best to build a panel that is diverse across many dimensions; I typically include at least one man, at least one woman who presents as "conventionally feminine," several international students, and, minimally, one student who identifies strongly with a spiritual tradition. My hope, as I am sure is obvious, is to expose the students to as broad a range of feminist expressions as possible. After a semester of seeing me—a white, middle-class, middle-aged woman—representing feminism, I want to leave them with a deeper, more complicated sense of what "feminist" looks like. But what I find wakes them up most is not the racial, gender, ethnic, and religious diversity of the panelists, but the content of the panelist's messages. Students' ears perk up as one panelist describes her comfortable commitment to shaving her legs. When another panelist admits that she unapologetically loves slasher movies, they lean in. When a young married panelist shares that her husband takes out the trash and she does all the cooking, I see smiles and detect relief. It is the eroding of rules that define feminism that magnetizes the students. Their fear of feminism, in part, is a fear of not doing it right, of not being able to completely line up their values with their daily living. Of course, if feminism does not at least prod its adherents to make changes in their lives congruent with feminist values and push others to do the same, feminism slips from a social movement to a lifestyle, I fear, but the spirit of embracing contradiction as a practical reality (and even a sly recruiting strategy) does hold promise.

Everyday Feminism: Feminism You Can't Keep in a Box

This vision of an inclusive, interconnected, yet contradictory feminist movement challenges the boundaries of what does and does not constitute feminism. Logically it seems a diverse and at times incoherent movement that stimulates diverse social change action that may fall outside a conventional second-wave definition of feminism. Many third-wave narratives tell of women doing feminism without knowing or labeling it as such. Third-wavers often cite mothers as feminist role models for the ways they lived their lives every day, even though the mothers themselves would never have labeled themselves or their activism "feminist." For example, in an essay that explores black feminism, mental illness, and motherhood, Siobhan Brooks writes about the women "who organized against welfare cuts, and drugs in their neighborhood, for better housing and daycare, who would never call themselves feminist." In her story of surviving sexual harassment, Kiini Salaam attributes her resilience to her parents, whom she considers to be feminists even though they never uttered the word. She ascribes them this identity because they "injected the same power, pride and self-governance into [her] sisters' upbringing as they did in [hers]."[33]

Everyday feminism also includes daily acts of resistance that may or may not be enacted under the feminist banner. Lamm explains that for her, "for now, the revolution takes place when I stay up all night talking with my best friends about feminism and marginalization and privilege and oppression." Cecilia Balli describes this aspect of feminism as

> the feminism that I can't keep in a box, that I can't fully articulate. It is the feminism that is more disposition than discourse and that doesn't even call itself feminism. It is the stubborn self-instruction that despite the setbacks, I have to keep trudging forward; the quiet assurance that even if things went terribly wrong, I would survive. This feminism measures achievement in

everyday victories; a sister's new job, a redecorated room, a clean credit report. It celebrates the company of cousins and aunts around the kitchen table and cherishes our opportunity, finally, to complain, to laugh, to sing.[34]

This approach incorporates all kinds of feminist action, from traditional protests and marches to the everyday feminism described earlier. Though it may seem to stretch the definition of feminism rather thin, the point here is to expand feminism to embrace the mundane daily actions that, in the aggregate, constitute an accomplished life led with purpose and strength. Young feminists are using the second-wave mantra of "the personal is political" as a stepping-stone to understanding the needs and direction of the movement. As JeeYeun Lee explained in her reflection on her Asian American identity in a racist, tok-enizing society, by finding a language and starting to explain her experiences, she began to "link them to larger societal structures of oppression and complicity" and "find ways to resist and actively fight back."[35]

Concerning the four themes in the aggregate, what conclusions can we draw about what's important to third-wave feminists? What is evident is the replacing of strict boundaries and reductive divisions, choosing fluidity over rigidity (even if these characteristics are a fiction about second-wave feminism, as I discuss later). This desire for fluidity is often expressed via playful engagement with boundaries. Through the use of cyberspace—categorically a new development since the second-wave—and DIY (do-it-yourself) tactics, third-wavers play with appearance, gender, sexuality, and more. "Girlie Feminism," so dubbed by Baumgardner and Richards, is the attachment to "disparaged girl things [such] as knitting, the color pink, nail polish and fun." The pierced, lipsticked, and coiffed body, the wardrobe that expresses the full spectrum of gender, and the sex-positive drawer filled with dildos, all become activist sites of third-wave articulation. To quote Reger: "In contemporary feminism, the everyday (and everybody) becomes the palette for third-wave political action."[36]

But wasn't the personal famously political in second-wave feminism? Yes, of course, argues women's studies scholar Lisa Maria Hogeland, who contends that so-called third-wavers seem to have missed the point of personal transformation by reducing it to little more than a narcissistic politics of identity: "The personal is political was meant to argue that politics construct our lives at home, as a way of breaking the public/private barrier in our theorizing—it was never meant to argue that our lives at home were our politics."[37]

Missing the point may be the consequence of an impoverished sense of femi-nist history. Many critics of third-wave feminism call attention to the seeming lack of historical understanding that obscures the third wave's indebtedness to the second wave. Orr, for example, admonishes some third-wavers' "misremem-bered, or at least extremely narrow, version of history."[38] Are third-wavers con-versant with the history of second-wave feminism—its intramovement debates and fractures, the varieties of feminist theories and practices that flourished throughout the era? Through third-wave eyes, the second wave looks like a monolith—little more than a middle-class white women's movement concerned with a narrow range of issues addressed by an uninspired stable of tactics. It is easy to reject such feminism—so partial, so limited. But the plentiful social histories and analyses of the U.S. women's movement since the 1960s document again and again the richness of the movement manifested in innumerable campaigns, alliances, and organizations, making it impossible to name not a feminism, but feminisms, not a women's movement, but movements.[39]

Like Orr, Reger detects continuity between the waves when she traces connections between yesterday's feminist activism and today's: "While the sense of 'play' may be new, many of the 'playgrounds' are not."[40] For example, many second-wavers, particularly radical and lesbian feminists, zeroed in on diverse sexualities to counter the hegemonic heteronormativity that limited self-expression. Like third-wavers, they used clothing to make political statements (and certainly, this was true in the first wave as well, when Amelia Bloomer pushed for dress reform in the form of less restrictive clothing).[41] But these connections are not, it appears, often acknowledged, leading some second-wavers to feel as though their past labors are negated. Celebrated feminist Gloria Steinem articulated this sentiment most famously when she admitted that reading the words of third-wave feminists left her feeling "like a sitting dog being told to sit." Dicker and Piepmeier explain the dynamic thus: "Although claiming the presence of the third-wave has been an exuberant act for young feminists, it has been seen by many in the second-wave as profoundly alienating, an act of amputation. This perception is not entirely inaccurate; many third-wave feminists perceive the second-wave as a movement to which they don't want to belong, and they are not quiet about these feelings. According to many third-wavers, second-wave feminism is repressive and restrictive, and this is one reason that the third wave has had to break away and formulate new ways of being feminist."[42]

The implication that second-wave feminism failed to address the realities facing women erases the activist successes that, for example, built domestic violence shelters; pushed for the removal of homosexuality as pathology in the *Diagnostic and Statistical Manual of Mental Disorders*, the mental health field's bible; rewrote sexual assault statutes; and instituted sexual harassment policies in schools and workplaces. As Kimberly Springer points out, the implication of an out-of-touch second-wave feminism also serves to erase the labor of women of color who worked during and between the so-called waves, articulating the very intersectional analysis so championed by third-wavers and initially developed by second-wavers.[43]

Nevertheless, the hard distinctions between the waves persist. Why? Why do third-wavers, in particular, work so hard to differentiate, even exaggerate the distance between "us" and "them"? Henry explores this divide by interrogating the mother trope that characterizes so much interwave discourse. She finds that deploying a "matrophor" (an apt term coined by Rebecca Dakin Quinn) "suggests that there is something to be gained from turning feminism—and often feminists—into 'mothers' ...; [this matrophor] appears to embolden feminism's 'daughters,' granting them authority and a generational location from which to speak."[44] We all want, goes the logic of the matrophor, to separate from our mothers, believing that we, the smarter, savvier daughters, can and will do it better. But what are the ills of the mother, exactly? It is hard to locate a coherent critique except those stated in the abstract (too rigid, too narrow, too dogmatic) and those that point to demographics (too white, too middle class). The mother-daughter dynamic seems to depend on a monolithic characterization of the second wave, a rendering of feminism's past that mandates detachment, like that of the developmentally appropriate adolescent splitting from her parent. It is a story of dissociation on the path to independence, regardless of the veracity of the daughter's allegations against her mother.

The third wave's reductive treatment of the second wave is not unique to the women's movement. The process of maturation, the eclipsing of one generation by the next, may require a less-than-savory rendering of the past to facilitate the growth of the future. Certainly, the LGBT (lesbian, gay, bisexual, and trans) rights movement has experienced similar stresses and strains. The homophile organizations of the early twentieth century were supplanted by more assertive, vocal, and strident lesbian and gay activists, many radicalized by the dawn of the U.S. AIDS epidemic.[45] Today, transgender rights activists and queer theorists have again transformed the movement, rattling some old-guard activists and energizing and validating others. Joshua Gamson inspects the intramovement conflict in the LGBT movement through an analysis of the debate over the use of the word "queer." The debate over the emotionally freighted word with the painful past pits assimilationists, who have no use for an epithet, against those who reclaim "queer" with liberatory pride. But this is not a new struggle. Social movement participants are always jockeying, as Gamson puts it, "over who is considered 'us' and who gets to decide." And so, "despite the aura of newness ... not much appears new in recent queerness debate; the fault lines on which they are built are old ones in lesbian and gay (and other identity-based) movements."[46]

While a young activist's finding her voice is crucial, her doing so at the expense of movement solidarity and effectiveness is cause for concern. Rather, some say, a historically informed, holistic, and forward-looking perspective on the feminist movement holds more durable promise. It is the challenge of the next generation of feminists, equipped with their values of inclusion, multiplicity, and contradiction and their emphasis on the everyday, to move forward with, not in spite of, the history that shapes them. "The challenge for contemporary feminism is to take a look at past waves (or at least campaigns, organizations, protests, and sit-ins) and uncover the relationship between the past and the present," Reger writes. "Feminist history provides insight into the roots of current ideology and strategy."[47]

———

The story of the emergence of menstruation as a feminist preoccupation, a rather invisible chapter in feminist history, offers an opportunity to take up Reger's challenge to "uncover the relationship between the past and the present." Menstruation's invisibility complicates this endeavor; indeed, menstruation's uneasy place in the private and public spheres reflects a detachment from the body that is common to countless people. When a girl has her first period, our response, as historian Joan Brumberg shows, is rarely an invitation to welcome her new womanly status ("Time for a party!"), but more commonly a knowing smile and a scramble for menstrual products ("Time to go to the drugstore!"). This may be one of the first lessons a woman in training learns about her body and its place in the social order: "It will do things that we need not speak of. You will relate to it primarily as a consumer."

When women ignore their bodily processes or, worse, recognize them merely as problems whose solutions are available only through consumerism, internalized oppression takes over. I am suggesting not that detachment from the body—from what Adrienne Rich calls "its bloody speech"—is women's fault, but that when women participate in the silences around menstruation, they allow others to speak for them.[48] Today it is rarely women who define the meaning of their bodily processes and take self-directed action to experience them in ways that are healthy, sustainable, and, for some, enjoyable and renewing. Menstruation is one of those bodily processes, but it is not the only one. Pregnancy, birth, breastfeeding, menopause, nutrition, exercise, health care, even sexuality across the lifespan, are similarly co-opted by social institutions and discourses. Not those who inhabit the bodies, but physicians and other health-care providers, along with corporations, pharmaceutical companies, and their marketing machines, shape our cultures of embodiment. And there are those who feel strongly that feminists—whatever their wave—must resist such co-optation.

CHAPTER 2

━━∞∞∞━━

Feminist Engagements
with Menstruation

I know no woman—virgin, mother, lesbian, married, celibate—whether she earns her keep as a housewife, a cocktail waitress, or a scanner of brain waves—for whom her body is not a fundamental problem: its clouded meaning, its fertility, its desire, its so-called frigidity, its bloody speech, its silences, its changes and mutilations, its rapes and ripenings. There is for the first time today a possibility of converting our physicality into both knowledge and power.
—Adrienne Rich, *Of Woman Born*

In *The Curious Feminist*, Cynthia Enloe asserts the need to develop a *feminist* curiosity, which begins with "taking women's lives seriously."[1] This essential and focused attention, she argues, is not simply an act of valorization, but an earnest reckoning with all kinds of women in all kinds of places and times. When we take women's lives seriously, we attend to the gaps and the absences in women's lives, and accordingly to their consequences. Close attention to menstruation, for example, can reveal much about cultural values and identities. Some feminist analyses already point to the wide-ranging social and personal implications of this biological event. For example, Karen Houppert's 1999 journalistic exposé of the FemCare industry lays bare the stealth (her word) tactics used by purveyors of tampons and pads to teach women the importance of cultural practices that, she asserts, rely explicitly on the consumption of products, in spite of their questionable safety profile. Building on Houppert's work and situating a critique of corporate control of the menstrual body in an existential feminist framework following Simone de Beauvoir, Elizabeth Kissling argues that "the social construction of menstruation as a woman's curse is explicitly implicated in the evolution of woman as Other." In fact, "menstruation does not make woman the Other; it is because she is Other that menstruation is the curse." Kissling analyzes the representations and discourses surrounding menstruation because menstruation refracts the status of women in contemporary culture. Alice Dan (cofounder of the Society for Menstrual Cycle Research, an interdisciplinary network of menstrual cycle researchers and activists founded in 1979) and her colleague Linda Lewis chime in: "The menstrual cycle not only is a central aspect of women's lives, but it also offers a model to researchers who want to understand relationships between mind and body, and between social meanings and individual experience."[2]

Despite menstruation's centrality, even our language fails to represent it adequately, as linguist Suzette Haden Elgin knows. When she invented a woman's language in 1984, Láadan, she included words that capture women's diverse experiences of embodiment: to menstruate, to be pregnant, to menopause. For example, "husháana" means to menstruate painfully; "desháana," to menstruate early; "weshana," to menstruate late; and—my favorite—"ásháana," to menstruate joyfully. In Láadan, a woman can "azháadin"—menopause uneventfully.[3] Láadan constructs an alternate reality that challenges the dominant cultural narrative. But feminists such as Elgin are relatively rare; indeed, feminist scrutiny of the politics of menstruation pales in comparison to feminist engagements with other aspects of women's lives.

The feminist response to political issues centering on menstruation has largely been avoidance. Alice Dan remembers a reputed biologist and founder of the Association for Women in Science who declined an invitation to give a keynote talk at the first interdisciplinary menstrual cycle conference in 1977 because "she believed it was unwise to focus on things that make us different than men" because "they will use it against us."[4] I presume she was cautious of going "down there"—into the dark and dangerous essentialist territory where women are reinscribed forever as linked to (and thereby trapped by) their bodies. Not much has changed. Just a few years ago, when I submitted the title of a talk sponsored by feminist faculty at a liberal arts college in the Midwest, I was asked to eliminate the word "menstruation" for fear that it would cause trouble for the college's press office.

But there is another kind of trouble: feminist priorities in a universe of seemingly endless gendered injustices. One of the first questions after I gave a talk on this book in progress was posed to me by a well-respected historian: "Your work is really interesting, but with all the other issues women face, why choose menstruation? Aren't there more important things for feminists to worry about?" I take her question seriously. Certainly, with a Supreme Court stacked with conservatives chipping away at women's reproductive rights; a cultural climate that still blames women for their victimization in spite of staggering rates of domestic violence, sexual assault, and sexual harassment; the booming exploitation of women throughout the world as enslaved domestics and sex workers; and the atrocities of wars and occupations and their gendered consequences for women, there is much work to be done. Menstruation can seem a trivial concern. But I contend, following the menstrual activists who educated me, that close inspection of menstrual culture and its hazards is not detached from these concerns. Indeed, menstrual activists assert that menstruation's uneasy place in both the private and public spheres reflects a detachment from the body, as well as the long reach of hyperconsumerism, at the root of so much human suffering.

For any number of reasons, menstruation not only has languished on the margins of feminist inattention generally (or at best been masked in polite language), but also has eluded the focus of social researchers. Observes sociologist Laura Fingerson: "It is odd that such an integral and routine event in women's lives, which has significant implications for women's health and well-being over the life course, not to mention the salience it holds in adolescence, has generally been ignored in social research."[5] A body of scholarship exists, but it is limited. Some of the most popular texts on the subject are anthropological studies of non-Western and traditional societies, such as Thomas Buckley and Alma Gottlieb's 1990 *Blood Magic: The Anthropology of Menstruation*, Chris Knight's 1991 *Blood Relations: Menstruation and the Origins of Culture*, and Penelope Shuttle and Peter Redgrove's often-cited 1988 *The Wise Wound: Myths, Realities, and Meanings of Menstruation*.[6]

When it comes to menstruation, the fascination seems to be with faraway people in another time—their bizarre customs, their menstrual huts, their menarche rituals. Graduate student Sophie Laws felt this bias when she proposed a dissertation on contemporary British men's attitudes toward menstruation and met with questions like, "Why not look at what other cultures are doing?" Laws stood her ground and later published her study as *Issues of Blood: the Politics of Menstruation*, a work that delves beneath the surface of what she calls "menstrual etiquette" to conclude that, largely, contemporary ideas about menstruation derive from men. She argues that such androcentric cultural dictates specify that women should behave in public settings as if they did not menstruate, denying the monthly hormonal changes that accompany their cycles throughout the fertile years. Men can waive these rules in certain situations, such as in the context of heterosexual sexual contact. "What we have is a menstrual etiquette," Laws writes, "part of a larger etiquette of behavior between the sexes, which governs who may say what to whom, and in what context. Women are discredited by any behavior which draws attention to menstruation, while men may more freely refer to it if they choose to. Thus the etiquette expresses and reinforces status distinctions."[7]

This mandate is even more uncompromising for women of color, who are held to a racialized standard of "sexual respectability," a concept Evelyn Higginbotham developed in her historical study of black Baptist women, *Righteous Discontent*.[8] The "bloody speech" of women who lack white privilege is marked as especially dirty, disgusting, and "unladylike." Women of color, already socially constructed in white supremacist culture as "animalistic" and "out of control," can approximate legitimacy only if they deny their embodiment.

Containment and Negativity

The mandates of menstruation, that is, the relegation of menstruation to the domain of the personal and private, are consistent with the detachment from the body commonly practiced in contemporary Western societies. As the philosopher Elizabeth Grosz wonders:

> Can it be that in the West, in our time, the female body has been constructed not only as a lack or absence but with more complexity, as a leaking, uncontrollable, seeping liquid; as formless flow; as viscosity, entrapping, secreting; as lacking not so much or simply the phallus but self-containment—not a cracked or porous vessel, like a leaking ship, but a formlessness that engulfs all form, a disorder that threatens all order? I am not suggesting that this is how women are, that it is their ontological status. Instead, my hypothesis is that women's corporeality is inscribed as a mode of seepage. [9]

Leaky, liquid, flowing menstruation—a uniquely female experience associated with sexuality—is constructed as a shameful form of pollution that must be contained. Menstruation, then, is constituted as a problem in need of a solution.

The demarcation of the dangerous, problematic female body is evident perhaps most eminently at the time of menarche, the first menstrual period. In contemporary Western societies, girls face a paradox surrounding menstruation: They are often congratulated for entering womanhood, and they are instructed to keep their new status a secret.[10] While it may be true that menstruation is discussed more openly today, research shows that the impact of menstruation—in both Western and non-Western societies—remains largely negative.[11] Although experiences differ widely, one metastudy of the literature that examines emotional reactions to menarche concluded that most women experience negative and sometimes mixed emotions at the time of menarche.[12] For example, in a study of the reactions to menarche of women from thirty-four countries, most participants reported negative emotions, and a mere few mentioned either positive emotions or a combination of negative and positive emotions.[13] In a study of Zimbabwean women, professional women and domestic workers alike most commonly reported fear and worry associated with their menarche.[14] Still another study reports that Chinese adolescents met their first menstruation with negative reactions.[15] The negativity attached to menstruation, some say, discourages authentic engagement with one's body. For instance, Ros Bramwell links women's doubts about their capacity to breastfeed with negative perceptions of their own bodily fluids, including menstrual blood:

> Negative representations of menstrual blood may arguably undermine attempts to promote breast milk and breastfeeding. For instance it may affect women's

confidence, and lower confidence in ability to breastfeed has been shown to
predict failure to meet one's goals for breastfeeding. Moreover, such negative
constructions of female bodily fluids may produce negative attitudes which
are little changed by positive information about the benefits of breast milk
which de-contextualize the milk from the female body, and fail to address the
underlying negative constructions of female body fluids. [16]

It Wasn't Always This Way

Given the persistent strength of dominant menstrual consciousness—the negativity, the silence, the shame—and the varied sources of power that reinscribe
such constructions, making assumptions is tempting. Many of us presume that
the constellation of cultural prohibitions against open discussion of menstruation
and even, in some cultural contexts, menstruating women themselves is as old as
menstruation itself. But the history of the menstrual taboo, for example, is curious.[17] To begin, it did not appear to be a feature in classical Greece (in spite of significant medical attention to menses). It wasn't until biblical times that ancient
Jewish tribal societies began to see the menstruating woman as a source of pollution. Scholars of menstruation often cite this passage from Leviticus: "And if a
woman have an issue, and her issue in her flesh be blood, she shall be put apart
seven days: and whosoever toucheth her shall be unclean until the even."[18]

Characterization of menstruation as "the curse" in Western societies did not
emerge until the nineteenth century. In the Middle Ages, the semantically pleas-
ing word "flower" was commonly used to signal menstruation. Other metaphors
referenced regularity (such as "period" or *règles*) or the menstrual cycle's relationship to the moon. In seventeenth-century England, menstruation was construed as the requisite shedding of an excess of blood. This process, per se, was
not pathologized, although menstrual fluid was considered unclean and foul.
Rather, the failure of the process of excretion was seen as a symptom of disease,
a concern that inspired the development of remedies designed to restore normal
menstrual flow.[19]

As historian Joan Brumberg shows, the medicalization of menarche dawned
at the close of the nineteenth century as medical authority eclipsed maternal
influence. Previously in Western culture, the beginning of menstruation was
a maturational event, "a marker of an important internal change in a girl—
specifically, her new capacity for reproduction."[20] But during the Victorian era,
male physicians intervened in what had been a female domain and assumed the
role of expert, taking over the definition and treatment of menstruation, which
increased the demand for physician services. The new medicalized know-how
took the form of health and hygiene guides. The American Medical Association's
1913 pamphlet *Daughter, Mother, and Father: A Story for Girls* is a prototype of the
kind of "safe script" (as Brumberg describes it) middle-class Americans handed

to their daughters. Central to this script were the particulars of sanitary protection, which quickly materialized as markers of modernity, class privilege, and respectability. (The first disposable menstrual pads were introduced at the end of the nineteenth century.) Thus menstrual etiquette increasingly engaged autonomous teens as consumers.

In the wake of World War II, mothers, who had been a fixture in menstrual product advertisements, faded away. At that point, the industry began marketing directly to young girls and cleverly cultivating brand loyalty. Innovative and ubiquitous, the industry's advertising campaigns were (and remain), according to Andrew Shail and Gillian Howie, "the most explicit and loudest form of discussion of the menses" and have effectively "secured the tenacity of 'protection' as a set of ideas adhering to the menstrual (and so the female) body, a discourse which demarcates the female body as a danger to itself." This dangerous female body demanded an acute fixation on the embodied presentation, a preoccupation that became and remains the stuff of American girlhood. "When contemporary American girls begin to menstruate," as Brumberg concludes, "they think of hygiene, not fertility. That is the American way, and it is taken for granted—as if it were part of the natural order."[21]

Disciplined and Docile, Yet Resistant

The natural order, of course, is a powerful imaginary. To better understand it, I draw on Michel Foucault's conception of power as diffuse and aleatory. Foucault argues in *Discipline and Punish*, his critical treatise on the development of modern incarceration, that power is more regulatory and normalizing than sovereign and monarchial, and it is exercised at the level of daily life.[22] Thus, following Foucault, feminism as a theory and practice of social change needs to be concerned with how power over the body operates at both individual and collective levels, asking not only how the individual is disciplined but also how the collective is regulated. Because resistance operates at both levels, research that interrogates oppositional discourses and practices must engage questions of specific individual strategies as well as of collectivized contestations surrounding menstruation, historically and in the contemporary context.

After Foucault, bodies, as material sites of contention, exist as canvasses upon which cultural priorities and preferences are inscribed. With the exception of the few bodies typically deemed acceptable—those coded in mainstream culture as thin, taut, able-bodied, young, and white—bodies are always problematic and in need of correction through the vehicle of consumption. In the case of menstruation, the problem is its very existence; the solution is to render the process invisible by containing the menstruating body or, increasingly, eliminating it altogether through cycle-stopping contraception, that is, menstrual suppression. We can theorize this containment using another of Foucault's central contributions, that of the "docile body," a theoretical construct that allows us to conceptualize the internalization of certain cultural priorities fundamental to the maintenance of both seen and unseen power structures.[23] Foucault argues that in the industrial context, bodies are "produced" to function efficiently in the military, the factory, and the school. To illustrate, he discusses Jeremy Bentham's "panopticon," a nineteenth-century French prison design that enabled constant inmate surveillance. Such unrelenting observation "induces in the inmate a conscious and permanent visibility that assures the automatic functioning of power."[24] The process of each inmate's internalizing the perspective of the jailer is replicated in women's internalization of the misogynist gaze. Drawing on Foucault, one feminist philosopher, Sandra Bartky, examines a series of "disciplinary practices" that constitute femininity—gesture, posture, movement, and bodily comportment. Through these, Bartky illustrates how women are directed, simultaneously by everyone and by no one in particular, to transcend nature and correct every bodily "deficiency."[25] Women, under relentless scrutiny, hold themselves to a standard of normative femininity preoccupied with youth and beauty.

But some, like Monique Deveaux, take issue with Bartky's application of Foucault to women's embodiment. For her, Bartky fails to acknowledge the adage "Where there is power, there is resistance." Deveaux finds Bartky's conception of women's interactions with their bodies "needlessly reductionist," eliding the complexity of women's experiences (based on differences in age, race, culture, sexual orientation, and class), as well as the choices women make—often explicitly against the very standards of femininity. For Deveaux: "Bartky's use of the docile bodies thesis has the effect of diminishing and delimiting women's subjectivity, at times treating women as robotic receptacles of culture rather than as active agents who are both constituted by, and reflective of, their social and cultural contexts."[26]

Indeed, the menstrual activists at the center of this book provide a very concrete example of the kind of resistance Deveaux imagined (and Bartky omitted). They consciously resist docility, realizing their agentic subjectivity. Their engagements, rooted in different and sometimes conflicting feminist ideologies, attempt to reframe menstruation. In other words, they pay attention to the body's "bloody speech" in the interest of social transformation. And consistent with Foucault's formulation of power as shifting and unstable, the targets of menstrual activism vary, producing a movement rich in tactics.

Pathologizing Menstruation

In her now-classic study on the uses of gendered metaphor in scientific discourse, *The Woman in the Body*, Emily Martin demonstrates how metaphors of mass production that emerged during the industrial revolution championed values of quantity and efficiency and cast female bodily processes as failed production. Medical texts applauded the male body for producing a continuous supply of sperm while the female body, equipped with its total supply of eggs at birth, simply ages and degrades. In Martin's view: "Menstruation not only carries with it the connotation of a productive system that has failed to produce, it also carries the idea out of production gone awry, making products of no use, not to specification, unsalable, wasted, scrap. However disgusting it may be, menstrual blood will come out. Production gone awry is also an image that fills us with dismay and horror."[27]

Thomas Laqueur also explores the representation of menstruation in nineteenth-century medical discourse, finding the characterizations of menstruation in at least one influential account "redolent of war reportage." To illustrate his point, Laqueur quotes Walter Heape, whom he describes as "an immensely influential researcher on reproductive biology, not to mention a rabid antifeminist." Heape described menstruation as "a severe, devastating, periodic action [which] leav[es] behind a ragged wreck of tissue, torn glands, ruptured vessels, jagged edges." Laqueur draws on such characterizations to show the effort doctors put into establishing what he calls "the artifice of sexual difference."[28] Without difference, after all, the case for the subordination of women is undermined.

Provocatively, Martin challenges conceptions such as Heape's by imagining menstruation from a feminist standpoint, at times playfully modeling knowledge production in resistance to patriarchal medical authority. Rather than the purpose of the menstrual cycle being the implantation of a fertilized egg—clearly not the aim of every fertile woman, especially those actively using some form of birth control, Martin "can see no reason why the menstrual blood itself could not be seen as the desired 'product' of the female cycle, except when the woman intends to become pregnant."[29] (This concept will resonate for any woman who has dreaded an unplanned pregnancy and breathed a sigh of relief when her period began.)

A few other feminist accounts similarly interrogate the ideological dimensions of the menstrual experience. Situating menstruation as "at once an object of medical ideology" and "a cultural event intimately bound up with larger questions of the place of women in society," Louise Lander, in *Images of Bleeding*, argues from the standpoint of second-wave women's health-movement participants. In this view, menstruation became "an important focus of medicine's social function as agent of larger social forces in keeping subservient groups, such as women, where they belong." Historically, says Lander, such rules have usurped women's own sense of what their menstrual cyclicity means to them (implying, it seems, that an authentic embodiment can precede language and ideology).[30] Instead, women have turned to medical authorities, namely physicians, rather than rely on their lived experience as authority. Menstruation has been used to prove women's inferiority and unsuitability for everything from pursuing a college education comparable to a man's (which could be ruinous to women's health) to being elected president of the United States or nominated to the Supreme Court (Oh, the dangers of PMS!).[31] Menstrual cramps were diagnosed as a symptom of neurosis, even after it was established that cramps occur only during ovulatory cycles.[32] When menstrual pain is not pathologized to justify women's subordination, it is trivialized and interpreted as "just in their head," psychosomatic proof of women's frailty and instability.

Researchers of the menstrual cycle, most notably the members of the international, interdisciplinary Society for Menstrual Cycle Research (SMCR), thus walk a fine line between views of menstruation as incapacitating and as inconsequential. Past SMCR president Sharon Golub addresses this tension in her 1985 edited collection *Lifting the Curse of Menstruation* when she echoes Laqueur: "Since the menstrual cycle is such an obvious difference between the sexes, correlates of the cycle are regularly raised as evidence of women's inferiority and many people believe that women are victims of their repeatedly cycling biological systems. . . . While arguing against the idea that menstruation is debilitating for most women, it is important for us to attend to the real problems that it may present. A majority of women do report unpleasant or uncomfortable symptoms associated with the premenstrual and menstrual phases of the cycle."[33]

FEMINIST RESPONSE TO PMS AND PMDD

Sorting out the real problems from those conjured up in the service of sexism is difficult work. Take, for example, premenstrual syndrome (PMS), identified and documented in 1931 by Robert Frank as "premenstrual tension" and renamed "premenstrual syndrome" by Katharina Dalton in 1953, as Kissling reports in *Capitalizing on the Curse.* An excess of 150 PMS symptoms have been identified and subdivided into the categories affective, cognitive, behavioral pain, and physiological, according to Kissling, for which more than 327 treatments have been suggested to date, though most lack evidence of clinical effectiveness.[34] The long reach of the PMS self-help industry is apparent in a list of recent publications: *Taking Back the Month: A Personalized Solution for Managing PMS and Enhancing Your Health; PMS: Solving the Puzzle—16 Causes of Premenstrual Syndrome and What to Do about It!; PMS: Women Tell Women How to Control Premenstrual Syndrome; Vinnie's Cramp-Kicking Remedies: And Other Clever Cures for PMS, Bloating, and More; Once a Month: Understanding and Treating PMS* (sixth revised edition); and *Unmasking PMS: The Complete PMS Medical Treatment Plan.*[35] The book titles represent PMS as a mystery, a conundrum, and an invasion into a woman's life. And indeed, many women do complain of severe pain, debilitating nausea, and disabling mood changes, including feelings of depression, irritability, and sadness. The challenge for feminists concerned with women's health has been how to acknowledge the realities of

PMS without capitulating to, as Lander puts it, "updated underpinnings [of] the Victorian image of woman as inexorably ruled by her reproductive cycle, made unfit by her cyclicity for full participation in commerce and public life."[36] Blaming biology for the behavior of women (or men) is a classically antifeminist position, but so is the failure to take women at their word and validate their experiences.

Acknowledging this tension, some feminists have forged ahead with critiques of PMS that reveal the misogynist social construction of the syndrome, as Lander does here: "The personality traits that tend to emerge premenstrually in PMS sufferers—anger, aggressiveness, irritability—are precisely those characteristics that women, especially wives and mothers, are not supposed to possess. Women are supposed to be docile, patient and altruistic; thus being otherwise is pathological."[37]

A number of critics have focused on the newest diagnosis, that of Premenstrual Dysphoric Disorder (PMDD), which first surfaced in mental health discourse in 1985. Considered an extreme variation of PMS, PMDD is a mood disorder linked with the luteal phase of the menstrual cycle, which occurs between ovulation and menstruation. Key symptoms include irritability, anger, and depression much more severe than that associated with PMS. In 1993, after a protracted battle within the psychological community, PMDD was included in the American Psychological Association's *Diagnostic and Statistical Manual of Mental Disorders—DSM-IV(R)*—a handbook mental health clinicians rely on to classify and diagnose mental illnesses. While the manual lists PMDD only in the appendix (thus designating it a research category, not a diagnostic label), a code number is attached, permitting clinicians to use it as an official diagnosis. According to Kissling, however, "there is still no known etiology for PMDD and no empirical evidence that it exists," a position voiced by members of SMCR who expressed strong opposition to the inclusion of PMDD in the *DSM(R)*.[38] Nonetheless, the development and marketing of psychotropic drugs to treat PMDD has proceeded unabated. Prozac, repackaged in feminized pink and purple and sporting the trade name Sarafem, is now prescribed to women complaining of PMDD. The old drug's new name, many critics assert, was chosen in a transparent attempt to destigmatize the antidepressant.[39] Only six months into Sarafem's launch in 2000, the number of prescriptions sold reached eight million.[40] Kissling takes umbrage at Sarafem's campaign slogan "More like the woman you are," contending: "The clear implication here is that the premenstrual self is inauthentic [an idea Kissling credits to *Listening to Prozac* author Peter Kramer]; mood swings, irritability, and bloating aren't real feelings. Women must take psychotropic drugs to find their authentic selves and to suppress those unpleasant, unfeminine feelings that get in the way of their responsibilities. Medication can restore women to the 'Eternal Feminine' that characterizes the absolute Other."[41]

No More Periods?

While disagreements over the pathological consequences of the menstrual cycle fester, some researchers and clinicians now construct the normal menstrual cycle itself as problematic, viewing it as an obsolete biological process easily eliminated through cycle-stopping contraception. In 2003 the FDA approved Seasonale, an oral contraceptive that taken continuously for ninety days reduces the number of a woman's periods to four every year. Approved in 2007, Lybrel is an oral contraceptive taken 365 days a year that completely eliminates menstruation. Lybrel eradicates even the withdrawal bleed that occurs during a woman's cycle on standard oral contraception (a bleed that is mostly water, some blood, and a tiny bit of uterine lining, since oral contraception prevents the growth of uterine lining).[42]

Numerous health-care professionals, including feminist health activists and others who research the menstrual cycle across the lifespan, are not ready to deem menstrual suppression a risk-free health-care choice, especially for healthy women who consider continuous cycle-stopping contraceptives "lifestyle drugs." For example, the SMCR sounds a note of caution in a 2007 position statement posted on its website:

> While we recognize that cycle-stopping contraception may be useful for some medical conditions (such as severe endometriosis), we caution against its use as "a lifestyle choice" until safety is firmly established. Historically, nasty surprises with hormonal therapies for women (e.g., heart disease and hormone therapy for menopausal women, the link between oral contraceptives and blood clots, DES, and various health problems) have taken years to surface. Additionally, when any medication is evaluated for healthy women, the potential risks should be weighed more heavily than in situations when medication is considered to treat a disease. Menstruation is not a disease. [43]

Even before the FDA's approval was made public (in the context of debate between ardent supporters of suppression and opponents calling for more research), the mainstream press grabbed the story. Yet the popular media fail to provide a balanced account of the issues at stake, according to a content analysis by Ingrid Johnston-Robledo, Jessica Barnack, and Stephanie Bye of twenty-two U.S. and Canadian popular magazine articles about menstrual suppression: Advocates of menstrual suppression were quoted twice as often as opponents. The researchers were alarmed by the paucity of information regarding the long-term implications of menstrual suppression (sixteen articles) and the nearly uniform pathologizing of the menstrual cycle that characterized regular menstruation as an unnecessary inconvenience (nineteen articles). They concluded that popular press coverage of menstrual suppression is "inadequate" and "biased."[44] This is evidence, say some feminists, that menstrual suppression is less a blessing for women than a boon for business.

Emily Martin presciently focuses on menstrual suppression and the "alarm bells" she heard when first learning of the use of birth control hormones expressly to reduce the number of menstrual periods. Speaking of Seasonale, Martin offers the following caution: "Despite the obvious appeal [of menstrual suppression] we must wonder what the price of such fashionable convenience might be." She allows that "women for whom menstruation causes serious problems might welcome the cessation of their periods. But to make all menstruation pathological for all women goes far beyond the bounds of what we know and begins to sound like a scientific replacement for the idea that menstruation is dangerous and polluting. One has to wonder whether the virtual elimination of women's periods might make women's bodies appear more calm, steady, and predictable, in short, less 'troublesome.'"[45]

Some may argue that all feminists should support menstrual suppression as a clear expression of women's agency: If women don't want their periods, they shouldn't have to have them (comparable, of course, to pro-choice reasoning regarding abortion). Indeed, preliminary research suggests that if women are offered the option to do away with their menstrual cycle by a constant stream of estrogen, many will take it. A study conducted by Linda Andrist and colleagues asked women if they would be interested in totally eliminating their periods; 65 percent responded that they were not interested in menstruating every month, and one-third said they preferred to never have a period again.[46] If women can be released from the muss, the fuss, the discomfort, and the expense of managing their monthly flow, then *this* is women's liberation. But this reasoning presumes the following: Menstruation is necessarily a messy inconvenience without inherent value, and menstrual suppression is a completely safe health-care option that carries no risk. According to the SMCR and others, these beliefs are assumptions, not facts.[47] Still, feminists are hardly aligned on the suppression issue.

The Seasonale and Lybrel march toward FDA approval brought out a variety of feminist positions regarding the interface between technological innovation and embodiment. For instance, menstrual suppression is merely another in a long line of biomedical advances targeting women—advances that produce disparate reactions among those invested in resisting patriarchal constructions of women's bodies. Consider, for example, extant feminist debates over elective cesarean sections, surrogate motherhood and bioethics, and plastic surgery, which explore the extent to which women are agents utilizing developing technologies.[48] Feminist analysts ask: Are women empowered through the use of new technologies, or are they duped by the medical-industrial complex that exploits a particularly gendered set of assumptions about womanhood and motherhood?

On April 20, 2007, the *New York Times* carried a front-page story headlined "Pill That Eliminates the Period Gets Mixed Reviews," in which author Stephanie

Saul pointed to women's ambivalence regarding their periods as the reason the pill that stops menstruation has produced controversy. The article referenced Andrist and colleagues' research revealing that a majority of respondents were in favor of terminating their menstrual cycles, culminating in Andrist's interpretation of the study's results: "We don't want to confront our bodily functions anymore. We're too busy." Saul also interviewed filmmaker Giovanna Chesler, whose 2006 documentary *Period. The End of Menstruation?* screens across the United States and Canada. The aim of the film is to present a complex picture of the benefits and risks associated with menstrual suppression, for healthy and sick women alike. Chesler, believing that menstruation is not a disease and those who menstruate are not ill, reportedly said that women "don't need to control their periods for thirty or forty years."

But others, like *Reason* contributor Cheryl Miller, deem the call for more research and critique of antimenstruation a "strange feminist reaction," implying that feminists who do not support suppression are burdening women with the restrictions and stigma that menstruation brings. For Miller, it is all about giving women the choice to do what they will with their bodies. End of story. Her libertarian argument dismisses the sentiment (attributed to filmmaker Chesler) "that Big Pharma is a hotbed of misogyny," as well as the concern that menstrual suppression might ultimately undermine women's self-esteem, an opinion attributed to what Miller calls "granola-type" Anna C. Yang, director of the network of menstrual health advocates, the Red Web Foundation. In its conclusion, the SMCR position statement challenges reactionary standpoints like Miller's: "Finally, some have claimed that women should be 'free' to choose cycle-stopping contraception. But we firmly believe that authentic choice is only possible when accurate and comprehensive information is widely available."[49]

AND THEN COMES MENOPAUSE

As some women embrace the technologically assisted premature cessation of their periods—whether they see themselves as agents or objects—others, at the end of their fertile years, encounter the natural end of their menstrual cycles. The pernicious view that one's body is its own worse enemy combines with what feminist cultural critic Margaret Morganroth Gullette calls "age anxiety" to produce yet another market niche—the medical treatment of menopause.[50] The most popular treatment for what many perceive as the disease of menopause is so-called hormone replacement therapy (HRT). Promoted mostly to stem osteoporosis and heart disease (and other aspects of aging), HRT was embroiled in controversy when a large-scale study (the Women's Health Initiative, initiated by the National Institutes of Health) revealed that the hormone therapy (both estrogen/progestin and estrogen-only preparations) actually *increased* the risk of heart attack, blood clots, stroke, and breast cancer.[51] According to the National

Women's Health Network (NWHN): "The widespread popularity of hormone therapy (HT) in the United States is a triumph of marketing over science and advertising over common sense. Drug companies and many health care providers present menopause as a disease. In fact, it is a normal transition that occurs in all women."[52]

The NWHN is not alone in its criticism of the medical inclination to see menopause as pathology. Emily Martin asserts that this view not only is rooted in the interaction of ageism with sexism but also is "a logical outgrowth of seeing the body as a hierarchical information-processing system in the first place" and the postmenopausal body as analogous to the "disused factory, the failed business, the idle machine." As the Boston Women's Health Book Collective in its most recent edition of *Our Bodies, Ourselves* states: "The hormone controversy also raises an important bioethical issue. Many of us believe that the standards for using unproved treatments on healthy populations should be more stringent than those for treating people who are ill and choose to risk something new as a possible cure. Menopausal women are healthy."[53]

If we don't choose to shut down the factory or the machine (read: the body), we must at least keep it tidy. More urgently, the body—a dangerous entity—must be protected from itself, according to our cultural logics. And it is here that the menstrual activists enter. They question the fundamental assumptions that constitute what Brumberg calls "the natural order" of menstruation, exposing what is deemed "natural" as a socially produced set of values that serve patriarchal and capitalist interests.[54] The activists subvert the precepts of the dominant narrative of menstruation and strive for an authentic autonomous embodiment. Their aim is to seize agentic menstrual consciousness from the docile, disciplined body and stimulate new ways of knowing and being that neither shame nor silence. This work has begun; in fact it has a short but interesting history that until now has escaped a systematic documentation. I turn now to this history.

CHAPTER 3

The Emergence of
Menstrual Activism

Because Deb's engagement with menstrual activism is nearly as old as the movement itself, I asked her to explain what led her to swim against the mainstream and
embrace "alternative menstruation" beginning in the mid-1970s and continuing
through the early 1980s.

> I remember we were getting into organic foods and healthy alternatives in
> cosmetics, with natural lotions and toothpastes, et cetera. There were a lot of
> feminist and holistic health books coming out right then, it was the height of
> the women's movement in ways, and *Our Bodies, Ourselves* was just out, and
> we would read books and magazines for sale at the co-ops. One of the books I
> bought there was *Hygieia*. I read in *Hygieia* we should not hide our blood in
> shame and told my girlfriend about it. She agreed it was feminist for us not to
> hide our blood in shame. Also, toxic shock syndrome had just hit, and women
> were afraid. [1]

The dawn of the feminist health movement, growing interest in natural
products inspired by the environmental movement, and an outbreak of a little-
understood and frightening infection led to Deb's transformation. She was not
alone. Beginning in the 1970s, increasing numbers of women began to question
the safety of menstrual products and, more fundamentally, the social construction of menstruation as little more than a shameful process. They cultivated a
critical menstrual consciousness. As some feminists reclaimed menstruation,
refusing to remain silent about a crucial women's health issue, they joined in
coalition with consumer rights advocates and environmentalists and pressed the
government and FemCare industry to attend to safety and, to a lesser degree,
environmental sustainability.

THE WOMEN'S HEALTH MOVEMENT
AND ITS CENTRAL RESOURCE

The women's health movement, the mother of menstrual activism, became "a recognizable force of social change along with the reemergence of the feminist movement in the late 1960s and early 1970s."[2] Into the 1980s, the women's health movement provided significant resistance to standard medical practice, namely the promise of scientific objectivity, the economic abuse of patients, and the norms of the doctor-patient relationship. Key to the movement is the foundational assumption that under the dominant medical system, women have lacked control over their bodies and therefore their health. In this view, the medical system, designed and serviced primarily by men, ignores women's unique bodily experiences and thus fails to provide women-centered care.

Many see abortion, which emerged as a key feminist issue in the late 1960s, as the lightning rod for contemporary women's health activism.[3] Indeed, the late 1960s and early 1970s were a heady time for abortion rights activists. In 1969 a group of Chicago women formed Jane, an underground abortion counseling service that later became an abortion service provider.[4] In 1970 attorneys Linda Coffee and Sarah Weddington filed a suit on behalf of "Jane Roe." The suit made its way to the Supreme Court, and in 1973 the ruling in the historic *Roe v. Wade* case declared abortion a fundamental right. In 1971, women's health activist Lorraine Rothman began promoting menstrual or period extraction using a crude device. She invented and patented the Del-Em to manually extract the contents of the uterus when a woman anticipates her menses, or up until approximately eight weeks from the first day of her last menstrual period. Some women used the Del-Em to abort very early pregnancies. As these examples represent, feminists were committed to securing access to abortion for women in need. They argued, as reproductive rights activists do today, that the right to choose if, when, and how to become a mother is fundamental to a woman's quality of life and, more generally, to her capacity to act in her own best interest.

Other aspects of women's health were coming to the fore at this time as well. Pioneering women's health activist Barbara Seaman published her groundbreaking *The Doctor's Case against the Pill* in 1969, a watershed moment for the generation of activists that emerged in the 1970s. The book linked oral contraceptives to cancer, heart disease, diabetes, and stroke and exposed the unethical use of poor women of color as testing subjects for contraception research. The resulting congressional hearings in 1970 led to an FDA mandate that all birth-control pills carry warning labels. This was the first time the FDA permitted consumer input as part of a drug's regulation. As an article in the *New York Times* noted: "Barbara Seaman triggered a revolution, fostering a willingness among women to take issues of health into their own hands."[5] Seaman's work inspired a new breed of women's health activists and cast a spotlight on reproductive health, exposing the potentially dangerous consequences of "scientific advances" for women.

But Seaman was not alone in asking questions about the best interest of women and their health. A collective of radical feminist women from the Boston area who shared a deep distrust of the medical establishment produced a pioneering body of knowledge that empowered women as agents of their own health care. This small group connected at a women's health seminar in 1969 and began discussing their experiences with doctors (mostly negative) and their knowledge of their bodies (mostly inadequate). They decided to form the Doctor's Group to research topics germane to women's health and share their findings, eventually creating *Women & Their Bodies*, a 138-page booklet published by the New England Free Press in 1970. The group quickly sold 250,000 copies of the booklet in New England, mostly through word-of-mouth advertising.[6]

By 1973, the newly formed and incorporated Boston Women's Health Book Collective (BWHBC), numbering twelve women, expanded the scope of the book and under contract with Simon and Schuster published the strategically retitled *Our Bodies, Ourselves*. This 276-page text openly and honestly broached unmentionable topics, including orgasm, the clitoris, the pill, and abortion. Known for its candid first-person accounts and graphic and realistic images of female anatomy and of women kissing, this book, too, was a success.[7] Now in its eighth edition, the book has sold four million copies and has been translated or adapted into eighteen languages, including Braille. It is estimated that the book has reached twenty million readers worldwide, demonstrating, as Barbara Brehm observes, the truth of the maxim "knowledge is power." The newest edition specifically targets younger women, say the writers, "while continuing to appeal to the readers loyal to *OBOS* across its previous editions."[8]

The Consumer Rights and Environmental Movements

In contrast to the explicitly feminist aspirations and goals of the BWHBC, the menstrual activism of the environmental and consumer movements revealed the influence of a more subtle brand of feminism on broader social issues. According to sociologist Robert Mayer, the "fragile, but enduring" U.S. consumer movement emerged in three waves. It surfaced at the turn of the twentieth century during the Progressive era, when food and drug safety and regulation of competition emerged as concerns in muckraker exposés of the impacts of industrialization. In the 1920s and 1930s, consumer access to objective information and consumer representation mobilized activists. In the 1960s the third wave of the consumer movement was stimulated largely by investigative writers who tapped into "a society of highly educated consumers whose expectations regarding quality of life were rising," including, I would add, women who used a feminist lens to analyze the factors that compromised the pursuit of their own health and happiness. While safety has always ranked as the movement's number one issue, in the 1970s the movement "dramatically expanded its conception of what constitutes a consumer issue."[9] This broadening definition set the stage for feminists to push past the menstrual taboo and publicly address menstrual care.

The reformist consumer movement typically accepted mainstream values and worked to protect the quality of life of consumers, registering grievances against industries that produce harmful products and devices. According to Mayer, movement activity peaked in the 1970s and declined in the Reagan era of the 1980s when the possibility of change through government action waned; it was then, as Mayer observes, that "the movement lost whatever grip it had attained on the government's regulatory apparatus."[10] But at least one arm of the consumer rights movement that focused on health issues achieved measured success during that decade, perhaps due to the change of leadership of Public Citizen, a celebrated national not-for-profit consumer advocacy organization that joined the feminist health movement to produce menstrual activist success.

Like the U.S. women's movement, the nation's environmental movement proceeded in waves. Journalist Mark Dowie, author of a searing critique of the movement, *Losing Ground*, identifies three distinct stages. The first, in the late nineteenth and early twentieth centuries, coincided with the closing of the U.S. frontier and tapped into a burgeoning conservationist and preservationist impulse. Fast-forward to the second wave in the mid 1960s, a brief era of environmental legislation, as well as a surge of grassroots enthusiasm, much of it generated by the 1962 publication of Rachel Carson's *Silent Spring*. Carson's book exposed the devastating effects on wildlife and human health of the indiscriminate use of synthetic chemical pesticides, most notably DDT. In 1970 activists held the first Earth Day, an event that many historians regard as the "temporal boundary between the conservation and environmental movements . . . herald[ing] a national commitment to a healthier environment."[11]

But while environmentalism continued to seep into the public consciousness, the Reagan administration and its environmentally hostile orientation abruptly halted success at the governmental level, mirroring the barriers faced by the consumer rights movement. Attempts to find common ground with conservative national environmental organizations and corporate entities distinguished environmentalism's third wave, in the 1990s. Contemporary critics of the movement characterized it as little more than a "vast, incredibly wealthy complex of organizations dominated by a dozen or so large national groups."[12]

Other critics pointed to environmentalism's conceptual shortsightedness, including some feminists who cited the mainstream movement's failure to adequately address women's concerns. From their frustration with a fundamental dualism at the heart of the movement, that is, the positioning of the self in opposition to nature, a new wing of the environmental movement emerged: ecofeminism. Ecofeminists champion the interconnectedness of life and assert that hierarchy is the result of binaries, particularly the "self/other opposition."[13] In 1983 the first collection of ecofeminist essays appeared. Titled *Reclaim the*

Earth: Women Speak Out for Life on Earth, it describes ecofeminism as both theory and practice and identifies as relevant a wide range of issues, including antinuclear activism, women and land rights, women and world hunger, and most notably the international women's health movement. The confluence during the 1970s and early 1980s of these interrelated social change movements—women's health, consumer rights, and environmental—led to the emergence of a critical menstrual consciousness.

The Emergence of a Critical Menstrual Consciousness

During the 1970s, three strands—the women's health movement, environmentalism, and consumer activism—began to slowly intertwine to produce menstrual activism.

Phase One: From Convenience to Concern

The 1970 *Women & Their Bodies* addressed menstruation only briefly in a list of many cultural taboos surrounding women's bodies. This lack of attention appears consistent with prevalent attitudes toward menstruation. Most women were using commercial menstrual products (pads became available in 1896 and tampons in 1934), and this publication reflected no resistance to the products or, more generally, to the menstrual taboo. At this time, the industry, aware of many consumers' frustration with the belts and pins necessary to keep pads in place, unveiled adhesive strips. In its 1971 product launch ad, Kotex depicted a fashionably dressed woman joyfully kicking a box of New Freedom pads. The copy reads: "Whee! They're flushable! Welcome to the beltless, pinless, fuss-less generation!"

The pollution attached to single-use products had not yet registered, perhaps because the environmental movement was just beginning its transition from a conservation-focused enterprise. Even feminists were slow to list FemCare on the hit list of products that harmed women. Instead, women's liberationists (as they were called at the time) criticized hyperconsumerism and the premium placed on feminine beauty, connected to what some activists called "instruments of torture to women." During the notorious 1968 Miss America protest—the first national action organized by second-wave feminists—protestors tossed such offending objects as high-heeled shoes, bras, girdles, curlers, and false eyelashes into their stylized Freedom Trash Can, but implicated neither tampons nor pads.[14] At this time, FemCare was synonymous with liberation.

Nonetheless, the dangers of the menstrual taboo certainly captured the attention of feminists in the early 1970s. In 1971 feminist art pioneer Judy Chicago dramatically articulated resistance to menstrual shame and secrecy in the shocking photolithograph *Red Flag*, a close-up shot of Chicago removing a bloody tampon from her vagina. The artist later remarked that many people, in a stunning display of menstrual denial, did not know what the red object was; some thought

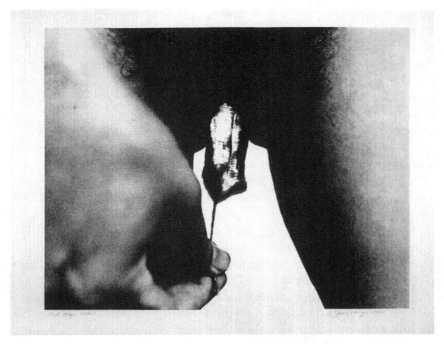

Figure 2. Judy Chicago, *Red Flag*, photolithograph, 20 × 24 in., 1971. © 2010 Judy Chicago/Artists Rights Society (ARS), New York. Photo © Donald Woodman.

it was a bloody penis. Chicago interpreted this ignorance "as a testament to the damage done to our perceptual powers by the absence of female reality." A year later in the installation and performance space Womanhouse, Chicago, Miriam Shapiro, and their collaborators explored gendered domesticity using the medium of a seventeen-room mansion in Hollywood, California. Womanhouse included Chicago's controversial and visceral "Menstruation Bathroom," a room liberally strewn with myriad used and yet-to-be used menstrual products. Chicago reinstalled "Menstruation Bathroom" in New York in 1995, and later in Los Angeles. Regarding the reinstallation, she remarked in an interview: "On this occasion, I was struck by two things—first that the range of sanitary products for women had grown enormously and second, the sense of shock elicited by this piece remained as potent as ever."[15]

The 1973 edition of *Our Bodies, Ourselves* addressed menstruation in a four-and-a-half page subsection under "The Anatomy and Physiology of Reproduction and Sexuality." The discussion did not touch on the politics of menstruation and quickly turned to product use, reflecting the view that menstruation was merely "a hygienic crisis."[16] Tampons and sanitary napkins were cited as "the most common method[s] of absorbing menstrual fluid," although "in a pinch there are clean rags and toilet paper." Without qualification, tampons were positioned as the most obvious and sensible choice of menstrual product: "Tampons are a convenience to many women."[17] Only two alternatives were introduced: the absorbent polymer Tassaway (a disposable menstrual cup) and "period extraction." *OBOS* acknowledged the Tassaway (pronounced "toss away"), first available in 1970, as an option but described it as potentially "difficult and messy."[18] The authors noted the second alternative, menstrual or period extraction, as experimental but "exciting for those of us who feel menstruation is a real burden."[19] The linguistic choice "those of us" suggested awareness that not all feminists or women's liberationists viewed menstruation as burdensome.

This inclusive language might have been a nod to one promenstruation feminist, Emily Culpepper, a student at the Harvard Divinity School and later a collaborator with the BWHBC. In 1972 Culpepper grew fascinated with menstruation while studying ancient religions. She first compared ancient Hebrew attitudes with contemporary attitudes toward menstruation and later explored ancient Zoroastrian menstrual taboos. This research inspired her to "help to create more positive, health promoting attitudes," which led her to encourage others to "look, really look, at menstruation, and see for [y]ourselves what it is."[20] Undaunted by her lack of filmmaking experience, Culpepper produced *Period Piece* in 1974. The ten-minute film included images and narratives associated with menstruation, such as a woman interrupting her work to change her tampon, and Culpepper's own first vaginal self-exam while menstruating. The film launched Culpepper's limited fame as a lay expert on menstruation, particularly menstrual attitudes, and she teamed up with members of the BWHBC to offer workshops locally and nationally, facilitating the raising of menstrual consciousness.[21]

In the same year that Culpepper produced her film, a small woman-owned business introduced natural sea sponges for use as tampons under the trademark Sea Pearls, expanding the number of options available to menstruators and suggesting that at least some women sought alternatives to conventional FemCare.[22]

Also in 1974, Barbara Hammer, the first openly lesbian filmmaker to explore lesbianism on the screen, made a ten-minute experimental film titled *Menses*.[23] Angry, raw, and unruly, the film explores a wide range of women's reactions to menstruation, an example of an early "talk back" to the FemCare industry. Among scenes of young naked white women washing between their legs, bleeding onto a white cloth (and then using it as a prop in a defiant dance), and participating in a simulated communion ritual involving a codeine pill and a cup of simulated menstrual fluid, we encounter women exiting a shop, their arms laden with menstrual products. One woman tears at a package of menstrual pads and furiously grinds them into the ground.

Around the same time, Emily Toth, Mary Jane Lupton, and Janice Delaney invited ten women to the first-ever "bleed-in," held in Lupton's bathroom. (The bleed-in was a play on the sit-in—a form of nonviolent direct action popular in the 1960s and 1970s that involved occupying a space in protest). The organizers were inspired by Chicago and other feminist artists, including Isabel Welsh, who created a thirty-minute taped collage of women talking about their menstrual experiences.[24] The organizers staged the event to stimulate their joint writing of a cultural history of menstruation that they eventually published in 1976. Their description of the bleed-in reveals their sense of breakthrough, of head-on confrontation with a powerful social taboo, softened with self-conscious humor:

> For the occasion, Mary Jane had decorated the bathroom with signs and symbols of menstruation. Large paper flowers were hanging from the mirror and the door. Stained pads (tomato sauce) were lying at random on the floor. Near the red wastebasket lay a pair of white pants with a red "Friday" stitched on the front and a telltale stain on the crotch, meant to recall the high school myth that a girl who wore red on Friday "had the rag on." Red yarn dangled from the rim of the door. On the wall was a piece of paper titled "Menstrual Graffiti," on which women wrote such witticisms as "We all need someone we can bleed on"; "Woman's place is in the bathroom"; and "Vampire to schoolteacher: See you next period."[25]

As some women challenged the menstrual status quo, others were responding to acute crises in women's health, among them the damage caused by a defective birth-control device worn inside the uterus, the Dalkon Shield. Despite knowing of the product's numerous safety problems, A. H. Robins Company continued its aggressive marketing campaign. The flawed device caused life-threatening pelvic infections for 235,000 women, two hundred spontaneous septic abortions, and thirty-three deaths. The injuries led to a recall of the product in June 1974, resulting in a famous class-action suit and numerous individual lawsuits.[26] This consumer crisis put feminist health activists on alert, setting the stage for growing skepticism about products that promised to alleviate women's reproductive health "problems." Two years after the Dalkon Shield recall, in 1976, Paula Weideger published *Menstruation and Menopause: The Physiology, the Psychology, the Myth and the Reality*, a pioneering book that sought to break the silence surrounding menstruation and the menstrual taboo as especially injurious to women's lives.[27]

In 1976 Delaney, Lupton, and Toth published their bleed-in–inspired book, *The Curse: A Cultural History of Menstruation*, which addressed the taboos, myths, rituals, and symbolism of menstruation from a feminist perspective. Devoting a full chapter, "Rags to Riches," to the menstrual products industry, they provided a succinct history of menstrual product innovation. The authors sought to dispel the myth that disposable and flushable products are biodegradable: Not only does the production process generate contaminated wastewater, but also tampon applicators wash up on beaches, while pads, tampons, and their packaging clog landfills, sewers, and water-treatment plants. This marked the first link between environmental degradation and conventional menstrual care.

While the chapter was largely historical and descriptive, Delaney, Lupton, and Toth's criticism of the industry was groundbreaking. The authors pointed out that "manufacturers have relied heavily on gimmickry to liven up sales," detailing how they "first created a need for scented products and then rushed to fill it." Explaining that menstrual fluid is odorless until exposed to air, the authors pointed out the uselessness of scented tampons, sold to a gullible public in spite of the FDA's "receiving reports that question the safety of these products," lamenting that "as in the case of sprays, such reports will probably have no effect on their success or failure in the marketplace."[28]

The authors also criticize sanitary napkins, "a breeding ground for bacteria," wondering why superior products were not available and complaining that no company had "made a tampon that a woman with a heavy flow can wear with complete security." However, while Delaney, Lupton, and Toth sought to expose the sexist root of the menstrual taboo and questioned the safety and necessity of menstrual products, they stopped short of a comprehensive anticapitalist critique of the industry that profited from that taboo. Indeed, in the chapter conclusion they sound grateful: "The manufacturers for the most part serve their customers well. They supply a product for which a real need exists, and they look hard for ways to improve it."[29]

In the 1976 edition of *OBOS*, the view of menstrual products remained static. Tampons and sanitary napkins were still noted as the most common choices, but the menstrual sponge was mentioned too. After a brief discussion of how the sponge worked and where to access it, the text returned to tampon use in words nearly identical to those of the 1973 edition. The diaphragm was introduced as an internal menstrual fluid collector and the Tassaway and menstrual/period extraction continued to be mentioned as alternatives. While making more options realistically available to consumers may have been an aim, these alternatives were included without a critique of dominant menstrual care options. A more trenchant criticism of the industry and its products was on the horizon, however.

On September 26, 1977, *Time* magazine ran a story titled "Women's Movement under Siege" that claimed the 1,500 delegates to the National Women's Political Caucus shared the impression that the women's movement was "faltering." This was a discouraging year for feminists, *Time* asserted. Citing the Supreme Court ruling that stopped the use of Medicaid funds for abortion services, the ERA's falling three states short of ratification, and the increasing might of the radical Right, it painted a dismal picture of beleaguered feminists sending up the white flag.[30]

But for menstrual activists, energized by nearly a decade of feminism's second wave, 1977 was a busy year. BWHBC members Esther Rome, a founder of the collective with an avid "scientific and feminist interest in the anatomy and physiology of sexuality and reproduction," and Emily Culpepper produced the brochure *Menstruation*. Available on request from the collective, its content departed significantly from the text included in *OBOS*. According to BWHBC cofounder Norma Swenson, the brochure, printed in red ink, was conceived as "a feminist challenge to the wretched inserts which came in tampon packages."[31] The brochure began: "Menstruation is a normal, usual, healthy occurrence for many years of a woman's life"; it went on to challenge "standard medical views" and devoted a full page to menstrual product use titled "What to Use for the Flow." This section acknowledged that "there are many ways women in different cultures have handled their menstrual flow," marking the first time the collective had contextualized and historicized menstrual management. Pointing out that "sometimes [women] didn't use anything" and "since earliest times" had made their own tampons and pads from available materials, the brochure acknowledged that "in *some* cultures women use commercial sanitary napkins and tampons."[32] The discussion quickly shifted to menstrual sponges (which women have "recently . . . rediscovered"), with a brief mention of the diaphragm, and included a caution to women to avoid deodorized products because of possible allergic reactions.[33] BWHBC's first challenge to the FemCare industry, the brochure echoed the critique of Delaney, Lupton, and Toth to "beware of possible problems with 'new, improved' tampons or napkins."[34]

Simultaneous with the BWHBC's release of its brochure, the Society for Menstrual Cycle Research held its first conference, legitimizing the menstrual cycle as a worthy subject of scholarly research and perhaps establishing the field as a serious and viable concern for activists as well.[35] Also during 1977, distrust of the "feminine protection" industry began to surface in the form of rumor. Investigative journalist Nancy Freidman attributed an "asbestos in tampons" myth that still survives today to the work of one New Age health magazine and other unnamed "feminist publications" that "picked up the information and circulated it."[36]

Further evidence of this consumer doubt took shape in myriad forms. An informational sheet circulated circa 1978 by the Berkeley Women's Health Collective indicted tampon manufacturers for their use of various chemicals and cotton-rayon blends. Accusing tampon manufacturers of "ignoring requests for a list of all substances contained in each brand of tampon," the sheet cited many hazards associated with tampon use, such as shredded fibers left behind in the vagina, the prevention of draining and discharge, and overdrying.[37]

Also in 1978 Jeannine Parvati published her now classic *Hygieia: A Woman's Herbal*. The tone of the book was vintage late 1970s, hippie discourse infused with cultural feminism, a strain of feminist theory that valorizes women and their experiences, particularly those associated with embodiment. While Parvati focused on alternative means of dealing with one's monthly flow, she represented menstruation as a positive and powerful experience. In her chapter "On the Rag & Other Menstrual Rituals," she cited "the images, our body fantasies, our cultural myths and poor health" as barriers to what she called the "*ecstatic renewal*" that connects menstruation to female sexuality.[38] She also included a hand-lettered pattern for homemade reusable cloth menstrual pads. Parvati's book represented a paradigm shift.

Hygieia's illustrator, Tamara Slayton, became a fertility awareness consultant for the state of California and embarked on her own menstrual health work in 1978, adding her voice to the growing chorus of discontent. Inspired by an unplanned teen pregnancy that she was forced to hide, Slayton connected the "shaming of the fruit of the womb" with the pressing need for positive menstrual education for girls.[39] She founded a business, New Cycle Products, that a website dedicated to Slayton after her death from breast cancer described as manufacturing "the first natural menstrual Products—"Glad Rags.""[40]

In response to growing consumer awareness and concern, *Consumer Reports* released in 1978 the results of a survey of 4,500 tampon users, noting that "some women were worried that tampons could lead to vaginal or bladder infection, to erosion of the cervix, to hemorrhaging or to uterine growths. ... But our medical consultants assured us that neither tampons or pads are a hazard to health."[41] The contrast between this complacent tone from a key consumer-advocacy mouthpiece and cutting-edge feminist analyses of menstruation is striking. The feminist health activist critique of the medical establishment (which would question the assurances of "medical consultants") was missing from the *Consumer Reports* study. Not the first evidence of the difference in approach between feminist and consumer activists.[42]

The 1979 revised and expanded *OBOS* included new information drawn from the brochure created just two years earlier, but the depth and nascent skepticism were missing. This inconsistency is curious. It is possible that the brochure, distributed on request singly and in packets, was deemed a more appropriate medium through which to attack the FemCare industry. *OBOS*, heralded as evidence based and level headed, had quickly grown into a resource on which women could rely, a compendium of trusted information. Perhaps the brochure, with its limited circulation, was seen as a more appropriate place to do more confrontational activism.

Still, the 1979 *OBOS* did suggest that conventional products were not for everyone, a safe way to introduce criticism of the FemCare industry. While the authors acknowledged the popularity of sanitary napkins and tampons, this edition for the first time mentioned tampon incompatibility, the mismatch between a woman's menstrual needs and a particular type of FemCare product.

Without questioning the use of tampons, the text instructed users to accommodate their particular health needs by trying a slightly different product, with sponges, diaphragms, and menstrual extraction again suggested as alternatives. Absent were the caveat about deodorized or scented products, the suspicion about new and improved products, and the passage acknowledging cultural and historical differences in the ways women absorb their flow. But this more passive and accommodating approach to menstrual product use would undergo dramatic revision in the next edition of *OBOS*.

Phase Two: Enter Toxic Shock Syndrome

In 1975 Procter & Gamble (P&G) began test marketing Rely, a superabsorbent tea bag–shaped tampon containing chips of carboxymethylcellulose. Purportedly, one Rely tampon was so thirsty it could absorb a woman's entire menses.[43] After its test-market launch in New York, Judy Braiman, leader of a small consumer advocacy group called the Empire State Consumer Association, fielded calls from women who reported vomiting and diarrhea after using a free sample of Rely.[44] The year after P&G's regional launch of Rely, the FDA, coincidentally, began implementing new Medical Devices Amendments to ensure the safety and effectiveness of medical devices, including diagnostic products, which put the federal agency in a position to regulate FemCare products.[45] But it would take a lethal outbreak of Toxic Shock Syndrome (TSS) for the government to make such regulation a priority. Until then, FemCare was seen as a convenience, even among women's health advocates.

A rare but potentially fatal infection, TSS is caused by bacterial toxins, most commonly streptococci and staphylococci, that until the 1979 outbreak struck only minute numbers of people. Cases increased after P&G's introduction of Rely. Between October 1979 and May 1980, the Centers for Disease Control (CDC) received reports of fifty-five TSS cases and seven deaths; most were among women who experienced the onset of illness within a week following their periods. The TSS epidemic reached its peak in 1980 with 813 cases of menstrual-related TSS, including thirty-eight deaths.[46] By 1983 more than 2,200 cases had been reported to the CDC.[47] Under extreme pressure from the FDA and to avoid the imminent threat of a damning product recall, P&G "voluntarily" withdrew Rely from the market.[48]

P&G's handling of the outbreak angered many, including FDA scientists and especially the women and families touched directly by TSS. One high-profile case was that of Pat Kehm, a twenty-five-year-old woman who died of TSS while using Rely. The jury in the case found P&G liable for Kehm's death, claiming that P&G was aware of the health hazards associated with their product but failed to notify consumers, a claim P&G denied. Plaintiff's attorney Tom Riley stated in his closing remarks that "Pat Kehm died because Procter & Gamble let her die. . . . They were more concerned about their product than warning their customers." P&G was ordered to pay $300,000 in nonpunitive damages.[49]

At the very end of 1980, a team of CDC scientists published "Toxic Shock Syndrome in Menstruating Women" in the *New England Journal of Medicine* that established a superabsorbent synthetic tampon-TSS link.[50] Around this time, others pursued the cause of TSS (especially microbiologist Philip Tierno, now widely credited for solving the mystery behind TSS).[51] In response to intense media coverage and an outpouring of public concern, the FDA finally began to honor its mandate to regulate FemCare safety, although the targets of some its actions were suspect in the eyes of many menstrual activists. In addition to negotiating the Rely recall, the FDA upgraded tampons to a Class II medical device, meaning that tampons were now regarded as requiring more than "general controls" sufficient for safety and effectiveness and might even require "special controls" such as performance standards and postmarket survelliance.[52] At the same time, the FDA notified sponge manufacturers, mostly women-owned businesses, to stop distributing sponges for menstrual purposes. Menstrual activists regarded this move as a transparent (and sexist) effort to placate the public while leaving the true culprits—the commercial tampon manufacturers—relatively untouched.[53]

The health crisis precipitated by the outbreak of TSS provoked an outcry from feminist activists and garnered the concern and support of some members of the mainstream medical system, represented by the CDC. In its wake, the FemCare industry was forced to confront the potential hazards associated with its products, giving activists a foot in the door. Despite the clear need for federal regulations, however, the manufacture of safer femcare products remained voluntary, as the consumer activism that engaged directly with the federal agencies lost its strength. Tellingly, mainstream consumer advocacy organizations would be instrumental in producing the desired outcome.

In the same year as the TSS outbreak, Ralph Nader, author of the influential 1965 exposé *Unsafe at Any Speed: The Designed-in Dangers of the American Automobile* and founder of Public Citizen, ceded its leadership to Dr. Sidney Wolfe, who had previously headed up the organization's Health Research Group. Wolfe, described as "adversarial, unfair, self-serving, and someone who enjoys confrontation," emerged as a public and aggressive advocate for a number of health issues, including the standardization of tampon labeling.[54] But while Public Citizen ultimately won concessions from the government and industry that had eluded feminist activists, those very successes represented the degree to which feminist voices had shaped broad social concerns.

The ensuing years produced a wave of feminist activity on the part of industry and activists in the interest of making tampons safer. Tampon manufacturers, engaging in a bit of damage control, ceased using polyester foam in their products, but this was not enough to ensure their safety. In 1981 journalist Nancy Friedman published *Everything You Must Know about Tampons*, which discussed the tampon-TSS link and alternative products. Also in 1981, Rome and Culpepper revised and expanded their 1977 brochure *Menstruation* with a section titled "Report on TSS—March 1981." The newer brochure succinctly described TSS—its symptoms, possible cause, treatment and follow-up, prevention—and urged readers to "make corporations and those who fund research accountable to the public and especially women."[55] The BWHBC, spurred by an outpouring of consumer concern, was also busy pressuring the FDA to force manufacturers to label tampons with TSS warnings. In a letter dated June 22, 1981, the collective stated, "Last fall we received over 650 requests for information on toxic shock. We found that women wanted to know about TSS but had no readily available source of information besides continuous monitoring of the news media."[56] This letter served as important ammunition in negotiations with industry and government representatives in the next series of menstrual activist interventions.

Soon thereafter, the FDA requested that the Association of Testing & Materials (ATSM) convene a group consisting of tampon manufacturers, consumers, the FDA, and other interested parties to write a private, *voluntary* tampon standard (this in lieu of an FDA mandate of any kind). Beginning in 1982, BWHBC founders Judy Norsigian and Esther Rome together with Jill Wolhandler attended this group's meetings on behalf of consumers but quickly discovered an inherent clash of interests between industry and consumers.[57] In their article "Can Tampon Safety Be Regulated?" published in 1992 in *Menstrual Health in Women's Lives*, Rome and Wolhandler expressed their frustration with the ATSM group, which, "without producing any kind of standard," dissolved in 1985 after three years of virtual intransigence.[58]

While the FDA was unwilling to legally mandate safety and performance standards, it did issue a regulation in 1982 requiring a label on the exterior of tampon packages advising women to use the lowest absorbency tampons to meet their needs. But activists pointed out that this requirement was practically mean-ingless absent uniform absorbency descriptions across the industry (that is, one brand's "superabsorbency" might have been another's "regular"). Rome, Wolhandler, and nursing professor and reproductive health researcher Nancy Reame were among activists who initiated a campaign to standardize absorbency ratings. The tampon safety campaign captured more than the usual group of fem-inist health activists; it became a lightning rod for a broader alliance of consumer activists in the mid 1980s. The Reagan administration's aggressive efforts at dereg-ulation threw formidable roadblocks in the way of those who appealed to gov-ernment to protect the safety of consumers.[59] But the existence of intermovement collaboration strengthened those concerned with tampon safety. Drawing on the resources of the feminist health and consumer rights movements, especially the now more aggressive Public Citizen, menstrual activists pushed their agenda throughout the decade, even as the consumer movement lost steam and the envi-ronmental movement became increasingly institutionalized.

Illustrating that the tampon issue had attracted a broad constituency, a health advocacy group, Women Health International, in 1984 petitioned the FDA to develop a safety standard for tampons.[60] The edition of *OBOS* published that year reflected mounting concerns regarding tampons. Adapted from the 1977 BWHBC brochure, the section dealing with menstrual product use began: "Women in different cultures have handled their menstrual flow in many ways. Sometimes they don't use anything. Since earliest times, women have made tampons and pads from available materials, often washing and reusing special cloths or rags. Today, some women make them from gauze or cotton balls." The next sentence— "Most women use commercial sanitary napkins and tampons"—correctly reflected the trends in product use, but this time the chapter linked TSS to tampon use.[61]

This edition of *OBOS* included a more direct critique of the industry and the FDA, inspired by the gathering force of the feminist health movement, aided by consumer rights activists and other groups like Women Health International. Clearly, the TSS crisis transformed what had been whispered criticism into angry voices calling for change. For example, the authors' tone had sharpened regarding the lack of standardized absorbency ratings: "There is no premarket safety testing of tampons. Most research is done by the manufacturers who keep it secret. Although the law requires the U.S. FDA to set uniform standards for the safety and performance of medical devices including tampons, the agency has no plans to do so." This language, the strongest yet, portrayed the FDA as consciously neglectful. For the first time, *OBOS* politicized the sponge option, noting that the FDA did not approve the sponge for menstrual use and "concentrated on menstrual sponge distributors, all very small businesses, because of the political pressure on it to take some kind of action while the issue of TSS was prominent in the media." In a gentle nudge toward consumer activism, a footnote suggested to readers: "Report any tampon-related problems to the U.S. FDA. Write to the U.S. FDA to support uniform absorbency labeling and thorough safety testing for tampons. Even a few letters make a difference."[62]

Also for the first time, the 1984 *OBOS* evaluated menstrual hygiene practices from the perspective of women in wheelchairs, revealing that these women may be at special risk for the development of menstrual health problems (largely due to less frequent changing of tampons). Furthermore: "Those of us who have limited sensation in the lower part of our bodies or are confined to wheelchairs often find all of these methods either irritating or difficult to use. There is no satisfactory solution to this yet."[63] Despite the tone of resignation, the critique of available products as inadequate for some women opened up space for dissent in general and reflected the influence of the feminist health movement's analysis. (It also prefigures menstrual activist attention to movement inclusion, central to third-wave feminist ideology.) Finally, the caution from the 1977 brochure against industry innovations made it into the 1984 *OBOS*.

In the remaining years of the decade, activism picked up. *Lifting the Curse of Menstruation: A Feminist Appraisal of the Influence of Menstruation on Women's Lives*, edited by Sharon Golub, was published in 1985 and included a piece by Nancy Reame that discussed "menstrual problems related to hygiene practices" and repeated the consumer activist plea for "the need for a standardized absorbency test against which all brands can be comparatively evaluated." That year, Tamara Slayton founded the Menstrual Health Foundation, which was her answer to "the need for supporting women in gaining a deeper understanding and respect for their procreative cycles."[64]

In 1985 microbiologist Philip Tierno and colleague Bruce Hanna in the *Clinical Microbiology Newsletter* reported the results of their research on the superabsorbent synthetic tampon–TSS connection. Perhaps in response, Playtex and Tambrands voluntarily withdrew products containing polyacrylate rayon. At this time, tampons were losing their market share (tampon users declined from 70 percent of American women in July 1980 to 55 percent in December 1980).[65] Benefiting from this consumer shift, entrepreneur Lou Crawford began manufacturing a new product in 1987—the Keeper, a reusable menstrual cup made from natural gum rubber. The device, much like the defunct Tassaway, collected rather than absorbed the menses and for some menstruators was preferable.

During the same year Public Citizen began a tampon-absorbency warnings campaign that would continue through 1990. The group filed a lawsuit in federal district court to force the FDA "to issue a regulation requiring all tampon manufacturers to print, on the outside of every box, the numerical absorbency of the tampon along with the information that high absorbency puts women at higher risk of the often-fatal toxic shock syndrome."[66] This tactic of engaging the legal system was a departure from the approach of the BWHBC activists who chose to collaboratively interface with industry and government representatives and to organize consumers. That year, their letter-writing campaign—a favorite BWHBC organizing strategy—directly targeted the FDA and asked consumers to express their support of the standardizing terminology already on tampon boxes. Nearly three hundred letters were produced, 90 percent as a result of BWHBC's consumer alert.[67] But the era of mobilizing consumers to demand safer conventional products was coming to an end. A preoccupation with alternative products would soon eclipse the activist impulse to reform the industry, but not before key wins were scored, both in the United States and abroad.

Phase Three: A Success, a Failure, and the Shift to Alternatives

In 1989 Slayton published *Reclaiming the Menstrual Matrix: A Workbook for Evolving Feminine Wisdom*. The influence on her thinking of the feminist spirituality movement—an alternative to patriarchal religiosity—was apparent in Slayton's conception of menstrual consciousness as a matrix: "With menarche you meet your wisdom, and with your monthly bleeding you practice your wisdom, and then at menopause you become the wisdom."[68] But the biggest developments at the close of the decade centered on menstrual products. Also in 1989, Tierno and Hanna published in the *Review of Infectious Diseases* their research on the dangers of superabsorbent synthetic tampons. Their findings legitimized fear of tampons and helped create and maintain a market for alternative products in the United States.

However, the most significant stimulus for the alternative market was the result of feminist environmental activist success across the Atlantic. In the United Kingdom, Bernadette Vallely founded the Women's Environmental Network (WEN) and organized a national media blitz designed to enrage consumers and motivate them to take action against Britain's SanPro (from *sanitary protection*) industry's polluting methods. Vallely and fellow feminist environmentalists Josa Young and Allison Costello published the *Sanitary Protection Scandal*, which sold ten thousand copies in its first year, and the BBC aired a segment on the program *World in Action* detailing the hazards of chlorine-bleached paper products. According to Vallely, one in five people in the United Kingdom saw the show. The program drew attention to the effects of dioxin pollution and spotlighted the part it played in menstrual product manufacture.[69] Dioxin, a highly potent carcinogen, actually refers to a number of related chemical compounds known to be highly potent carcinogens and has been linked not only to cancer, but also to endometriosis and birth defects.[70]

British consumers, roused by the campaign, followed WEN's call to action. Women across the United Kingdom wrote more than fifty thousand letters to manufacturers and members of the British parliament demanding changes in the disposable paper-products industry. In a mere six weeks, all the major British sanitary protection producers had pledged to stop using the chlorine-bleaching process.[71]

But neither U.S. nor Canadian activists succeeded in replicating the British success. Vallely, who consulted Canadian activists inspired by the British campaign, concluded: "We failed to make much headway with the big companies compared to our British colleagues in WEN. Instead of engaging in a public debate about their products, the major corporations secretly agreed simply to ignore our campaign."[72] Why? Had the tripled forces of consumer rights, environmentalism, and feminist health weakened? The health-focused consumer advocates were still active, although without the benefit of the larger consumer rights movement to ground and support them. The environmental movement, according to Dowie, had "creat[ed] its own irrelevance by remaining middle class and white, pursuing 'designer issues' expedient to fundraising, focusing on Washington, lobbying the wrong committees, failing to move women and minorities into top jobs, building ephemeral memberships with direct mail, ignoring the voice of vast constituencies and, eventually—under the rubric of third-wave environmentalism—cozying up to America's worst environmental violators."[73]

In short, according to Dowie, the U.S. environmental movement sold out, a victim of its top leaders' unwillingness to build a powerfully confrontational movement and opting instead to play it safe. Movement leaders, he claims, insulated themselves, choosing not to reach into the grassroots, and existed largely as a "club of all white (and all but two) male CEOs."[74] Some who take a far less harsh view include Robert Musil, who points to the broader movement that

Dowie neglects. Dowie and others who angrily accuse the environmental movement of being too mainstream, too conciliatory, and too slow behave, says Musil, "as if only militancy mattered." Forgiving of what critics like Dowie might describe as the glacial pace of social change, Musil contends that "rapid changes, like the breakup of ice formations, are preceded by years of subtle shifts and signs that are easy to miss."[75]

If Musil is right, the growth of alternative FemCare businesses might have been the subtle change afoot. The proliferation of small, often women-owned companies suggests that a turn away from the industry was embraced as the best strategy to insure women's menstrual health. Natracare, a maker of non-chlorine-bleached pads and tampons that opened for business in 1989, traced its inspiration directly to the WEN campaign, citing both consumer needs and environmental sustainability. "The unconcerned response of the international feminine hygiene brands so appalled Susie Hewson that her immediate response was to undertake the development of her own tampons and pads with full concern for the health of women and the effect on the environment in production and at disposal."[76] Activists were growing increasingly concerned about the environmental burden of the production and disposal of single-use products.

In the United States, Lou Crawford began manufacturing the Version B Keeper, a smaller prechildbirth version of the menstrual cup, representing the beginning of a wave of alternative product development. Between 1992 and 1999, fifteen alternative FemCare businesses were founded, including all-cotton tampon and internal collection device manufacturers, reusable cloth-pad makers, and comprehensive distributors of various FemCare products.

Perhaps the most well known alternative FemCare business is the Canadian-based Lunapads International. Fashion designer Madeleine Shaw, weary of her "recurrent bladder infections caused by using tampons," turned to cloth pads but found the product a turnoff ("bulky, a hassle to use, and not particularly attractive"). Deploying her seasoned skills as a seamstress, Shaw designed her own pads with the "modern, urban woman" in mind. They were, Shaw says, "a hit" and were soon picked up by health-food stores. In 1995, Shaw opened her first store. Lunapads markets custom-designed pads, liners, panty liners, and panties made of soft cotton. The product palette is black, red, and pastels, some solids, some patterns. (One of my own Lunapads panty liners pictures fluffy white sheep against a soft pink background.) Shaw partnered with accountant Suzanne Siemens in 1999 and now reports approximately 20 percent annual growth in sales. Lunapads hosts a lively website, including a blog with an emphasis on green consumption, and a prominent social mission featuring Pads4Girls, a campaign to donate washable pad kits to girls in Africa.[77]

The North American response to the hazards of menstrual products (some documented, some not, but nonetheless real in the eye of the consumer) was a proliferation of alternative products. In 2006, I conducted an exhaustive

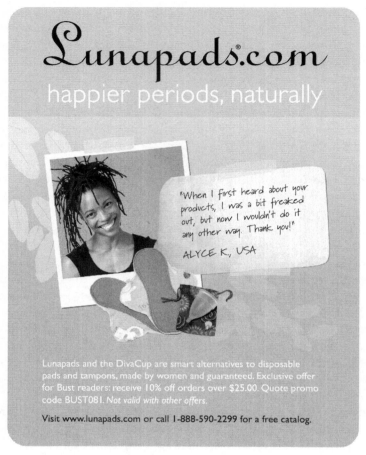

Figure 3. Lunapads print-ad campaign, 2008. Courtesy of Lunapads International Products Ltd.

English-language Internet search of FemCare business and located thirty to forty active alternative FemCare businesses based in the United States, Canada, the United Kingdom, New Zealand, and Australia. Nearly half were primarily web based (twenty-four of these responded to a brief questionnaire regarding company founding date and story, mission/vision, demographic served, and growth profile). But my count is apparently conservative. The website Cloth Pad Reviews in mid 2009 listed two hundred active cloth-pad makers and/or distributors and their websites.[78]

Perhaps this boom in the alternative menstrual product market, as opposed to a unified call for reform of the mainstream industry, reflects the hyperconsumerist context in which activism is necessarily embedded. The solution is not better products, but *more* products. Small numbers of activists did persist, however—consumer rights warriors who, in spite of a consumer movement in decline, forced the U.S. government to engage with product safety, even if in a limited way. For example, the judge in Public Citizen's case against the FDA ruled that the FDA had to publish a final regulation by October 31, 1989. The goal pursued by the feminist health activists associated with the BWHBC thus was ultimately achieved by consumer advocates, although the BWHBC had not withdrawn from the fight. In the summer of 1989, for example, BWHBC testified at congressional hearings on the Paperwork Reduction Act, protesting the ways government officials had delayed tampon regulation.

In addition to finally publishing regulations, the FDA addressed the tampon-dioxin risk that had electrified the U.K. public a year earlier, issuing a memo stating that the risk of dioxin in tampons "can be quite high."[79] But the FDA never forced the FemCare industry to change its bleaching methods, a step the industry took in response to consumer pressure. According to Jay Gooch, external relations manager of Procter & Gamble's Feminine Care division, the industry ceased using chlorine-intensive methods of bleaching in the 1990s.[80] Since then, "elemental chorine free" methods that employ chlorine dioxide, and "totally chlorine free" methods that replace chlorine with a bleaching agent such as hydrogen peroxide are in operation. Still, concerns remain. While the amount of dioxin produced using the "elemental chlorine-free" method is negligible, activists take a conservative position. For example, the Student Environmental Action Coalition (SEAC), which intermittently organizes a national Tampaction campaign, asks, Why risk the possibility of even *trace* exposure of a deadly poison, especially in the most absorbent part of a woman's body?[81]

The FDA did take action in another related area in March 1990, to the great relief of consumer and feminist health activists, formally implementing two criteria for tampon manufacturers: They had to advise consumers to use the lowest possible effective absorbency and standardize their ranges of absorbency. Around the same time, however, activists faced a setback when the FDA released a study that showed no cancer risk from dioxin in tampons. The data, supplied by the FemCare industry, did not include research design or testing of individual tampons or of how vaginal "dermal (skin) contact" might differ from other types of dermal contact.[82] That the FDA released a flawed study likely confirmed for activists their suspicion that the government agency was not genuinely committed to pursuing tampon safety and loosely veiled its allegiance to the FemCare industry. Menstrual activists of the next generation would express distrust of the FemCare industry (and the state charged with regulating it) and wage campaigns of DIY menstrual care.

True to its title, *The New Our Bodies, Ourselves*—the twenty-fifth-anniversary edition, published in 1992—significantly expanded its predecessors' treatment of menstrual products by including still more alternative options and introducing the potential health hazards associated with the industry's standard chlorine-bleaching process. For the first time, it listed rags as a material for homemade reusable pads. Included was the still accurate observation that "most women use commercial sanitary napkins and tampons," as was the list of possible problems associated with tampon use published in the earlier edition. Because the FDA in 1990 finally standardized absorbency ratings across the industry, *OBOS* elected to remind women only to "check the absorbency rating on the tampon boxes to help you select the lowest absorbency you need."[83] This directive marked the end of menstrual product safety activism by members of the BWHBC, fatigued and grateful to have finally won the labeling victory. The adoption of standardized absorbency ratings was a huge coup for menstrual activists. Furthermore, TSS had faded as the alarming issue it once was. As early as 1984, TSS incidences appeared to be dropping, due most likely to twin factors. First, average tampon absorbencies had been reduced.[84] Second, the issue had fallen off the radar of physicians responsible for diagnosing and reporting the infection.[85] Thus, flagging activist attention is understandable, though some committed feminists pressed on.

Among them, Esther Rome poured her seemingly endless energies into other women's health issues, including publicizing the dangers of silicone breast implants, raising awareness of sexually transmitted diseases, getting the first foreign language adaptation of *OBOS* off the ground, and writing (with Jane Wegscheider Hyman) *Sacrificing Ourselves for Love: Why Women Compromise Health and Self-Esteem . . . and How to Stop.*[86]

It took ten years for feminist health activists and consumer advocates— mobilizing angry consumers while congenially working with industry and government—to produce a rating system that was helpful to consumers. In "Can Tampon Safety Be Regulated?" Rome and Wolhandler in 1992 narrated their long uphill climb to improve the safety profile of tampons and concluded that "because women's health issues are not a research priority and because the FDA is limited in its effectiveness, product liability lawsuits will continue to be the single most effective way to make public results of manufacturers' proprietary research and to get questionable products off the market."[87]

In 1995 Rome died of breast cancer. Her impressive record as a women's health activist was celebrated at her funeral and in every subsequent issue of *OBOS*. Menstrual activist passion for *reforming* the FemCare industry in the interest of women's safety, however, died with her, but a new generation of activists emerged to advocate a radical transformation of the culture of menstruation. For them, reform of the FemCare industry was insufficient. Instead, activists variously pursued campaigns of radicalized consciousness and personal-level social change.

This wave of menstrual activists did not engage with government or industry or heed the advice of Rome and Wolhandler to pursue legal action but took a micropolitical approach to making change. The same trend operates in the environmental movement, now institutionalized and for some critics void of the energy it needed to effect real change. While Dowie may take a jaundiced view of U.S. environmentalism, I find his articulation of a key shift in the environmental movement reflected in the revitalized menstrual activism movement: "Grass-roots activists . . . seem to sense that much more is riding on the ability of the American environmental movement to reinvent itself than the success of a legislative strategy or the ability to prod scofflaw regulators with litigation; . . . what is clearly surfacing . . . is some much needed belly fire and a willingness to be audacious, confrontational, unpopular, and unphotogenic."[88]

Contemporary menstrual activists question the safety of the two main ingredients of tampons and pads—nonorganic cotton and rayon—and the bleaching process used in their manufacture. The problem with rayon, they say, is its abrasive properties. Rayon is a pulp product made of cellulose fibers, which can be left in miniscule amounts in a woman's vagina when she wears a tampon (especially after prolonged use). Fiber loss has been linked to vaginal ulceration and peeling of the mucous membrane, producing a breeding ground for infection. Furthermore, most cotton used in the production of tampon and pads is sprayed with pesticides. According to SEAC, cotton is one of the crops exposed to the highest concentration of pesticides.[89]

Contemporary menstrual activists still focus on the environmental devastation related to non-biodegradable, resource-intensive disposable products. Estimates vary, but if a woman uses five tampons a day for five days over thirty-eight menstruating years, she consumes and disposes of approximately 1,400 items. Some activists cite deforestation (rayon is a wood product), global warming, and marine pollution as additional environmental concerns. SEAC claims that annually more than twelve billion pads and seven million tampons are used once and thrown away, clogging our overburdened landfill sites. Further, the student organization asserts that an average menstruator throws away 250 to 300 pounds of tampons, pads, and applicators in a single lifetime; more than 170,000 tampon applicators were collected along U.S. coastal areas between 1998 and 1999.[90]

And activists point to the class dimensions of FemCare product use. FemCare is costly. Based on current product price in my market of Boston, an average lifetime supply of pads will cost the consumer around $2,200; of tampons, around $2,500. Most menstruators use a combination of products. Activists encourage women to avoid supporting a (mostly male-run) industry they regard as potentially hazardous both to women's bodies and to the environment and channel their resources elsewhere.

Throughout the three phases of the menstrual activism movement, challenges to the menstrual status quo transformed gratitude for menstrual products as conveniences into the skepticism that flourished in the wake of the TSS crisis. An alliance of feminist health, consumer rights, and environmental activists produced a vibrant movement across movements that refused to assume that industry and government would put women's best interests first. Today's menstrual activists can, if they choose, draw strength from and build upon this history.

————————

I turn now to the women and a few men who, in the present day, continue the tradition of menstrual activism. Just as up-and-coming environmentalists transformed the tactics of that movement in the last decade of the twentieth century, so did menstrual activists. But unlike many environmentalists, they did not cultivate collegial relationships with industry and governmental officials. Rather than initiating product liability lawsuits or pressing the government to more aggressively regulate the industry, they turned within. The contemporary movement has bifurcated into two wings, and their differences—both conceptual and tactical—are stark. One wing of the movement—the radical menstruation activists—promotes a dogged independence from convention. Taking their inspiration from punk-infused third-wave feminism, their style of resistance turns its back on corporations in the age of mega business and hyper consumerism. And their tactics are bold and confrontational. While many contemporary activists are not aware of the history that shaped their movement, their work today is (perhaps unwittingly) indebted to those who came before: a succession of artists, filmmakers, artists, authors, and activists inspired by feminism, consumer advocacy, and environmentalism, whose scrutiny developed a critical menstrual consciousness.

The other wing of the movement—boasting a longer history—is comprised of the feminist-spiritualists. They are the focus of the next chapter.

CHAPTER 4

～∞∞∞～

Feminist-Spiritualist Menstrual Activism

Nineteen-year-old Kami McBride was ill. It was 1981. When McBride sought medical advice, four different doctors told her she was simply manifesting the stress of a recent breakup, on top of college finals. While McBride acknowledged that stress is undoubtedly implicated in numerous health problems, she was not satisfied with this explanation. So she consulted a nurse practitioner and started to get different answers. Ultimately, a CT scan identified a tumor on her pituitary gland that McBride believed was linked to high dosages of estrogen-based birth control. During surgery to remove the tumor, the surgeon had to lift the front of her face to access the difficult-to-reach tumor. "When all was said and done, I had a different face than when I started," remembers McBride. Looking in the mirror at her altered nose and mouth, Kami McBride decided to pursue alternatives to hormonal birth control. She could no longer ignore the warnings attached to various birth control methods, even as many of her friends continued to take oral contraceptives and hope for the best.

But McBride did not want to surrender her body to medical experimentation or to settle for the convenience of certain birth control methods at the expense of her health. From that point forward, she became deeply interested in what she described as "the possibility to create a different experience of health" and placed herb study at the core of her exploration. Following the lead of holistic health advocates Tamara Slayton, Jeannine Parvati Baker, Rosemary Gladstar, Jane Bothwell, and Vicki Noble, McBride began to realize that is was possible to disengage from the dominant paradigm of health care that disenfranchises women and replace it with one that relies on ancient traditions, informed embodied self-awareness increasingly dubbed "body literacy," and holistic women-centered healing.

During her training, McBride had a second pivotal experience; this one awakened her to the links between the politics of women's health and the role of menstruation. During the lunch break of a class with herbalist Jane Bothwell, the students went swimming to beat the heat. When McBride declined an invitation to join everyone in the water because she was menstruating, her teacher encouraged her "just do what we do—bleed on the ground and wash it off in the pond." McBride recounts her epiphany: "I don't really remember anything else we talked about that weekend, but that statement rocked my world. Something cracked open and I saw that the shame around my blood was part of what kept me suppressed in general. . . . It was on this summer day that I realized how political women's health issues were." These two experiences changed McBride's life in profound ways. Since 1988 she has taught a full schedule of women's health classes. In 1994 she founded a herb school, which she built on a pristine patch of northern California forest. Her classes include a yearlong workshop, "Cultivating the Medicine Woman Within," and a three-day workshop, "Women's Wisdom: Health and Well Being for Menstruation, Fertility, and Menopause."[1]

McBride is a member of one of the two wings of the menstrual activism movement. I call the members of her wing "feminist-spiritualists"—menstrual activists who work to reclaim menstruation as a healthy, spiritual, empowering, and even pleasurable experience for women. Though the women I place in this category are diverse in their approaches, tactics, and philosophies, they coalesce around their common reframing of menstruation and effecting attitudinal change, woman by woman. Feminist-spiritualist menstrual activism is largely ideological and individualized, approximating what Anthony Giddens calls "life politics," a form of activism—rising out of late modernity's altered boundaries of social action—that concentrates on the everyday conditions of people's lives. In Giddens's formulation, life politics differs markedly from what he calls "emancipatory politics," more conventional quests for social equality. Key to his concept is the link between the self and the global context. Self-reflexivity does not occur in a vacuum but is connected to systems on the global scale: "Life politics concerns political issues which flow from processes of self-actualisation in post-traditional contexts, where globalising influences intrude deeply into the reflexive project of the self, and conversely where processes of self-realisation influence global strategies."[2] In other words, the global shapes the personal, and the personal shapes the global.

While the feminist-spiritualist menstrual activist project is certainly one of self-actualization, it stops short of reflexively making global connections, at least in the sense of authentic, strategic political engagement beyond the self. Rather, the feminist-spiritualist project is a modified, even truncated, form of life politics, which may in part explain the limited appeal of this style of activism. Relatedly, the lack of movement infrastructure may also compromise movement strength. I am aware of only one organization that connects activists and establishes visibility for this little-known movement: the Red Web Foundation, the Bay Area network of menstrual health advocates. This dearth of organizations is not unusual for new social movements focused on the microlevel or the everyday. But to have an impact, such movements must work to make the connection between individualized and collective action. Movement participants cannot languish in the personal. Rather they must turn "self-improvement [in] to world improvement."[3]

When I attended screenings of Giovanna Chesler's documentary *Period. The End of Menstruation*, which explores the debate over menstrual suppression, titters and groans from the audience greeted a scene that introduced a group of menstruation-positive feminist-spiritualists—a long shot of a circle of white women in flowing skirts dancing and singing an airy song, many with foreheads decorated with Hindu bindis (worn mostly by South and Southeast Asian women, bindis can represent religious affiliation or marital status, or serve a decorative purpose).The women in the clip were participants in one of McBride's "Women's Wisdom" workshops. They were reclaiming their bodies through mindful and communal movement and dance. The implication of the audience response was not uncommon—"Are those silly, freaky women still around?"— suggesting that such gatherings are historic throwbacks, trivial, self-absorbed, and hence inconsequential. But I've been *in* that dancing circle, and I know that the women take their participation seriously. Drawing on a rich tradition born in the late second wave of the women's movement, they believe that women-centered practices such as this produce momentous cognitive and practical shifts in women's lives, with far-reaching implications.

Kami McBride hopes the self-knowledge gained through such practices will have a ripple effect, passing from woman to woman to man to child and so on. There is reason to believe that they might. On her website, McBride lists a handful of testimonials she has collected over the years. One workshop participant enthuses, "This class has changed my life and now I see myself as a woman!" Another exclaims, "This is where the healing of our world begins," which implies that social change is possible through the development of body literacy.[4]

Some critics are quick to discount feminist spiritualism as a tired, dead-end strain of feminism, hopelessly stuck in the 1980s and oblivious to transformations in the U.S. women's movement, such as the emergence of third-wave feminism and its project of troubling woman as a unified and stable category. But the feminist-spiritualists are very much alive—still dancing, still chanting in their women-only spaces. It is difficult to assess how many individuals identify with this subgroup of feminists, but the large number of books on the topic attest to its popularity. These include Carol Christ's 1989 *Rebirth of the goddess: Finding Meaning in Feminist Spirituality*, Starhawk's *The Spiral Dance* (which celebrated two decades of publishing success with a twentieth-anniversary edition released in 1999), and Lucia Birnbaum's 2005 *She Is Everywhere: An Anthology of Writing in Womanist/Feminist Spirituality*.[5] The popularity of retreats, tarot cards, spiritualist music, and women's spiritual practice groups also supply evidence that feminist-spiritualists are numerous and widespread, at least in the United States. But if feminist spiritualism persists, profoundly impacting individuals qua individuals, why does it remain peripheral to the women's movement and, as a platform for social change, largely ineffective?

SPIRITUALITY, ESSENTIALISM, AND GENDERED UNITY

For feminist-spiritualists, the spiritual dimension of menstruation serves as a touchstone. For example, Joan Morais, author of *A Time to Celebrate: A Celebration of a Girl's First Menstrual Period*, told me in an interview: "All the menstrual activists I have met or read about have a spiritual aspect to their work." For them, menstruation is magical, mysterious, and powerful; it presents women with a unique opportunity to develop a self-awareness that puts them in charge of their bodies and their lives. Bernadette Vallely, founder of the British Women's Environmental Network, echoes this perspective: "Women menstruate and it isn't evil—and this is one of the *most* powerful times of her month—for magic, for darkness and depth, for contemplation, for earthy reality, for honoring bodily fluids."[6]

These women assert that menstruation is neither a curse nor a meaningless hassle. Rather, because it is a process unique to biological women, it connects them to each other and to the essential feminine within. For Barbara Hannelore, who has developed coming-of-age events for mothers and daughters, workshops on women's cycles, and menopause retreats, menstruation is "a prayerful state, a time of inner activism."[7]

For some, the essential feminine is expressed through female archetypes, especially the goddess in various forms. This, of course, is not new. In the 1970s and 1980s, the turn toward feminist spirituality attracted communities of mostly college-educated white women who, seeking positive changes in their self-understanding and personal lives, embraced and reclaimed age-old goddess traditions as a means to empower themselves and others. Writers such as Starhawk and Vicki Noble and feminist scholars such as Carol Christ, Merlin Stone, Riane Eisler, and Barbara Walker are especially central to this perspective. Psychotherapist and menstrual health educator Elayne Doughty thinks of herself "as a combination of Aphrodite and Baubo, the goddess of irreverence and vagina humor in my mind."[8] But most invoke the goddess" not as a spiritual force, but more generally as a feminine source of strength and guidance, an alternative to patriarchal constructions of a higher power.

Among contemporary menstrual activists, the archeological and mythological work of Marija Gimbutas is especially central because it reinterprets the place and functions of the goddesses of Old Europe and articulates the ways menstruation was framed in prepatriarchal, pre-Christian, and preindustrial contexts. Historically, asserts Gimbutas, women bled without shame, in synchrony with the moon and within communities of women.[9] Feminist-spiritualists endeavor to create contemporary contexts that reclaim this tradition.

In addition to their embrace of the goddess and ancient traditions, many of these feminist-spiritualists are indebted to the pioneering work of Tamara Slayton, who founded the Menstrual Health Foundation in 1984, ran her own cloth menstrual pad business, and wrote a small number of self-published books and pamphlets premised on her notion of a "menstrual matrix," a medium for women's enlightenment. Hannelore, a former student of Slayton, remembered that "her work with menstruation was always in this context of the larger meaning of things, considering the entire span of a woman's life, with menstruation as a matrix where a woman could go each month, into herself, to develop insight, perspective, and wisdom."[10]

Slayton's legacy within the feminist-spiritualist tradition is profound. Members of her Menstrual Health Foundation joined with the Menstrual Millennium (a group of twenty menstrual health educators and advocates organized by Helynna Brooke) to hold a first-of-its-kind conference, "Reweaving the Red Web," in 2003. The response to the conference led to the founding that year of the Red Web Foundation, to carry on Slayton's work with the women of the Menstrual Millennium. The organization thrives today, with a volunteer executive director, a four-member board of directors, a five-member advisory board, and thirty-six members. The group sponsored a public educational day, "In the Flow, Embracing the Cycles of Womanhood," in fall 2007.[11]

As a movement, menstrual activism, with its emphasis on what Giddens calls "life politics rooted in a collective definition of self," is among the new social movements that expand previous definitions of social activism.[12] Such efforts depart from movements historically fixated on class conflict and macrolevel social change, shifting the focus from structural change to a preoccupation with identity, culture, symbolic codes, and social relations.[13] The theory behind them legitimizes everyday life as a site of social change in contrast to, for instance, lobbying the state, protesting corporate decision making, or engaging in local electoral politics. Consistent with this focus, the feminist-spiritualists are not, for example, locked in battle with pharmaceutical companies who market so-called menstrual suppression to healthy women as a lifestyle choice. Nor do they organize school parents and board members to question corporate-sponsored menstrual cycle education. Instead, these menstrual activists target their actions at the level of the everyday, the intimate, and the individual. For them, social change happens slowly but profoundly, one enlightened and empowered woman at a time.

But our understanding of this form of activism is limited. As sociologist and ethnographer Ross Haenfler astutely observes, in spite of new social movement theory's ability to capture and interpret identity-based collective action, its failure to account for decentralized movements "has produced a vision of cultural challenge, lifestyle politics, and collective identity mediated through bureaucratic organizations."[14] Consequently, the lifestyle-based change work at the core of movements like menstrual activism, especially in the feminist-spiritualist wing, remains unexplained.[15]

THE ESSENTIAL FEMININE: THE GREAT UNIFIER?

A poem by Margaret Bertulli captures the sentiment particular to the feminist-spiritualist subset of menstrual activists, in which bleeding is a defining experience of womanhood.

> I bleed
> I bleed and I wonder
> "Will this be the last time?"
> I bleed, therefore I am
> "What will it be like?
> This cessation of menses?"
> The unequivocal end of child-bearing.
> And my womb, though childless,
> Will it feel the end of possibility?
> Perhaps.
> And then the unforeseen strength,
> Promised by gender and age, will come.
> The sureness, the wisdom,
> The spirit to sing my songs.
> I know this as all women before me have known.
> We know this as we smile at the moon[16]

This poem asserts that through menstruation, women know who they are and can feel whole and proud, that menstruation is fundamental to womanhood. Furthermore, as menstruators, women are linked to women of previous eras and, in the present, across class, race, and sexuality, and to some extent, age. In this view, bleeding is an essential woman's experience, a universalizing hallmark of fertility, sexuality, and identity. Lara Owen, in *Her Blood Is Gold*, echoes this view: "My period is a monthly occurrence in my life that I have in common with all women who have ever lived. Women living in caves twenty thousand years ago, priestesses in palaces in ancient Egypt, seers in temples in Sumer all bled with the moon."[17]

Owen's comment aptly represents the feminist-spiritualist position. Again and again, in workshops, in books, in newsletters, on websites and discussion boards, feminist-spiritualists reference menstruation as the common denominator of womanhood, a view that grows out of cultural feminism, a theoretical tradition of the late 1970s and early 1980s. One of many feminisms and sister to radical feminism and lesbian feminism, cultural feminism valorizes women in strategic defiance of the patriarchal constructions of women as subordinate and deficient. According to second-wave women's movement historian Alice Echols, cultural feminism emerged from radical feminism and distinguished itself through its "rejection of the left and confrontational politics."[18] It argues that such cultural devaluation of women is at the root of gender-based oppression and that gender equality will be achieved if so-called women's qualities (whether socialized or inherent), such as nurturance, empathy, compassion, and caring, are championed throughout society.

This active reassessment and valuation of such qualities, and thus of women themselves, spawns women-only (separatist) spaces where women can build community, avoid the influence of men, and cultivate the uniqueness of their womanhood. According to sociologist Barbara Ryan: "[Radical] cultural feminists consider patriarchy and masculine values to be the cause, not only of women's oppression, but also of capitalism, war, racism, and the destruction of the environment. Cultural feminism calls for a creation of a wholly redefined world, including change in linguistic, artistic, sexual, and symbolic conceptions of women." In the 1970s, because cultural feminism asserted an essential sameness woman to woman and women's fundamental difference from men, it temporarily unified the troubled feminist movement, at that time bifurcated along lesbian-straight lines. (Lesbian separatists, who believed a true feminist could not sleep with the enemy, were pitted against heterosexual feminists, who believed she could.) Echols argues that cultural feminism succeeded largely because it promised an end to this destructive impasse: "Cultural feminism modified lesbian feminism so that male values rather than men were vilified and female bonding rather than lesbianism was valorized, thus making it acceptable to heterosexual feminists." By 1975, after two years of struggle between radical feminists and cultural feminists, the latter eclipsed the former "as the dominant tendency within the women's liberation movement."[19] Cultural feminism's rule did not last long, however. Liberal feminism, an approach invested most generally in gender equity vis-à-vis women's access to historically male-dominated institutions, soon became the dominant face of the U.S. women's movement.[20]

But cultural feminism did not disappear. Psychologist Carol Gilligan, poet and theorist Adrienne Rich, sociologist and psychoanalyst Nancy Chodorow, and philosophers Sara Ruddick and Mary Daly have done much to keep it alive and well. Key to this feminist tradition is the belief that oppression is the consequence not of difference per se, but of a patriarchal hierarchy that denigrates and disadvantages women and the feminine qualities associated with them. Strategically, cultural feminists engage at the level of the personal, shaped by a radical view of embodiment in contemporary culture. Social change, it follows, does not begin at the institutional or structural level; rather, it builds from the grass roots to effect a revolution in consciousness. The cumulative effect of individual women claiming their power *as* women will erode the patriarchy. In *Of Woman Born*, Adrienne Rich offers specifics:

> Female biology—the diffuse, intense sensuality radiating out from clitoris, breasts, uterus, vagina; the lunar cycles of menstruation; the gestation and fruition of life which can take place in the female body—has far more radical implications than we have yet come to appreciate. Patriarchal thought has limited female biology to its own narrow specifications. The feminist vision has recoiled from female biology for these reasons; it will, I believe, come to view our physicality as a resource, rather than a destiny. [21]

Feminist-spiritualists in the menstrual activism movement readily adopted this framing of female biology as precious asset rather than liability. Kelly Rose Mason, cofounder of the Red Web Foundation, suggests, in striking similarity to Rich's sentiment: "When women and girls view their bodies as powerful sources of wisdom, profound healing occurs at the individual's physical, emotional and spiritual level."[22] Among the feminist-spiritualists, the very way one thinks about menstruation and responds to one's menstrual cycles is where the change happens. Greeting a girl's menarche with a party, for example, can create an important shift in menstrual consciousness that bodes well for her future self-acceptance and fulfillment. "The female attributes of sensitivity and increased awareness that are heightened during menstruation are gifts of the feminine that have been de-valued and instead need to be cultivated," Kami McBride said in our interview. "Currently, principles of violence and environmental devastation are rampant on the planet. It is the renewal and revitalization of the feminine principles of sensitivity, creativity and caring for life that can change the course of what is currently happening."[23]

One could view such essentialism as a trap, as I have argued elsewhere: Women's movements built on the ground of cultural feminism ultimately rein-scribe gender roles, working within rather than against the category woman as patriarchally constructed.[24] As Judith Lorber acknowledges (although she collapses radical and cultural feminism in her critique), cultural feminism's detractors point out that concentrating on gender as a unified category neglects other sources of oppression, such as those based on racial, ethnic, religious, sexual, and class differences.[25]

Nevertheless, for some white and middle-class women, especially those who find comfort in feminist spirituality, this wing of menstrual activism resonates. (Of the feminist-spiritualist menstrual activists I interviewed, 92 percent were white and 78 percent self-identified as middle or upper middle class.)[26] How does cultural feminism prescribe a transformed world if it relies on not only so-called essential qualities, but also a white and middle-class conception of womanhood? Owen's overdetermined connection to *all* women through the menstrual experience, quoted earlier, is an apt example of this universalizing tendency. While Owen is motivated by a quest for sisterly solidarity, her fantasy of unity obscures the reality of centuries of women who did not bleed for various reasons (such as illness, pregnancy, lactation, malnutrition, and atypical repro- ductive anatomy) and, more importantly, the great chasms between women dug by differences in social location. This blind spot in feminist-spiritualist men- strual activism may limit its appeal, particularly for women who do not focus exclusively on their embodied identities *as* women, such as women of color, whose lives are shaped at least as significantly by race. A false ideal of unity—the assumption that common bleeding connects all women—combined with an essentialism that fails to challenge the social construction of womanhood may explain, at least in part, why feminist spiritualism persists merely on the margins.

The Tactics of Feminist-Spiritualists

In November 2005 and November 2006, I participated in a Belly and Womb Conference, the brainchild of ALisa Starkweather, a women's empowerment trainer, teacher, and ceremonialist. Open to any woman or girl for a fee of $150, the daylong conference was held at a western Massachusetts intentional community.[27] Belly and Womb celebrated its eleventh year in 2009. On her website, Starkweather explains the purpose of the one-of-a-kind women-only event: "[It] has a wide 'birth' of reasons why it is important for us as women to gather and as women we have a distinct journey with our belly and womb. When we detest, reject or disown it we cut ourselves off from the very source that could feed us, nourish us and empower us to live more meaningful lives. It is a time for all women of all ages to meet one another eye to eye, heart to heart and belly to belly."[28]

At the first of the two conferences I attended, the day began with a ceremonial entrance into the main conference space. One by one, women snaked through a simulated birth canal to the sounds of chanting, the shaking of rattles, and the pounding of drums, inflected by Native American and West African traditions. The chant, written and recorded by Starkweather:

> You were born from a woman.
> Your mother has a name.
> No matter what your story with her,
> We honor the womb from where you came.[29]

At the top of the stairs, an octagonal room, also richly decorated, held two altars on its periphery (one was designated for women who have died as a result of belly- or womb-related illness, such as uterine cancer) and a series of tables containing literature, art, jewelry, and other products for sale, as well as brochures describing services such as breathwork and healthy sexuality classes. At the center of the room were bowls of water and fruit, seeds, and nuts for snacking. The group of about sixty mostly white women, ranging in age from late teens to late sixties, arrived together dressed in hues of red, some with bellies bared. A few wore bindis, some wore belly-dance skirts, one sported a tiara, and another displayed an elaborate weave of flowers in her hair reminiscent of Mexican artist Frida Kahlo's self-portrait headpieces. The women landed in the room wide eyed, some appearing a bit anxious, aware that this was not a typical conference. (I was ambivalent, feeling disengaged yet intrigued and moved—the perfect attitude for an ethnographer.)

The day offered a choice of workshops, two of which were held in the Red Tent. This stylized space served as a retreat and reflection space in the tradition of women-only bleeding spaces, such as those popularized by Anita Diamant's 1997 bestselling novel *The Red Tent*. The combined effort of several volunteers and bolts of cloth in shades of red, maroon, and pink had transformed a simple room into a virtual womb—warm, serene and deeply soaked in color—and I overheard visitors remark that it had become a special place, somehow ancient and holy. Regardless of menstrual status, all conference participants were welcome in the Red Tent to sit, rest, talk, and meditate in community with other women.

The Red Tent is comparable to the moon lodge of some Native American traditions, as well as to menstrual hut practices associated with various indigenous cultures throughout the world, spaces designed to seclude women during menstruation. According to anthropologists Thomas Buckley and Alma Gottlieb, "little is actually known of such episodes of seclusion," although the authors note that the custom has often been singled out by European and U.S. observers as evidence of women's subordinate status.[30] But, caution Buckley and Gottlieb: "We must consider the degree to which accounts of such seclusion have been inflected by the pride of missionaries and other colonists in putting an end to what they *perceived* as an evil, rather than by the lived experiences of women in 'menstrual huts.'"[31] That is, the menstrual hut may have served as sanctuary, rather than as a place to which menstruating women were shamefully banished. Other anthropological accounts challenge this interpretation.

Feminist-spiritualists regard the menstrual hut as a sacred space built in honor of women's capacity to menstruate. "[Red Tents are] going up all around us as we are reconstructing here on earth what we want to reclaim," writes Starkweather, who sees the proliferation as cultural change, a place of teaching and healing and for many, and a place of quiet contemplation.[32] As of June 2009, less than two years since she began actively promoting the idea, she reports, Red Tent Temples number more than thirty in more than twenty cities across the United States, one in the United Kingdom and others forming in Australia, Israel, and Bulgaria.[33] Starkweather's monthly Red Tent is held in her yurt in rural Massachusetts. Here, women serve women, facilitating the sharing of food, massage, artwork, stories, journaling, and music.

Critics like Sally Price question the accuracy of the menstrual hut model. Price notes in *Of Co-wives and Calabashes* that the Saramaka women of Suriname did not regard their menstrual seclusion as liberatory or pleasurable, but as a necessary duty. The celebrations began *after* women emerged from the hut. In a later essay, Price explores the possibility that "a false harmony has crept unperceived into the interpretation of one area of women's lives—the cultural handling of menstruation." She argues that the anthropological literature documenting menstrual cultures throughout the world has been misrepresented (and she includes Buckley and Gottlieb as offenders) "to advance a feminist agenda determined to locate examples of the possibility of menstrual joy" and asks: "Is it possible that some feminist writings have in effect, redecorated the menstrual hut?"[34]

In addition to the Red Tent, the Belly and Womb Conference included a healthful vegetarian lunch and dinner, belly-dance (or Middle Eastern dance) instruction, belly painting (by commission), and a community healing ritual. The latter was especially interesting. As Starkweather introduced the purpose of the ritual, she asked the assembled women: "Who among us has not accepted her body?" Remarkably, every one of the sixty-some women present—of all shapes and sizes—stepped forward. Silently acknowledging the pervasiveness of many women's struggle with negative feelings about their bodies, Starkweather then invited women to connect with their pain, their suffering, and their rage "felt down in the belly." In response, a few women emitted sounds, some guttural, some intelligible: "I am tired of being a single mother!" "I miss my mother!" "I am angry!" As more women joined in, a chorus of moans, screams, and sobs filled the room. The voices rose into a crescendo and then slowly died down. The background instrumental music (previously drowned out by the cacophony of women's voices) sounded soothing tones, and the women, exhausted and some still crying softly, waited for Starkweather to speak. After a period of silence, she talked of the crucial importance of doing this work of expressing ourselves honestly in a community of other women, and of the healing power of facing our truths "down in the belly."

In the late afternoon before dinner, at the Women's Council women shared stories of healing, triumph, and struggle. One woman joyfully disclosed her newly discovered sexual attraction to women. Another made an impassioned plea for vegetarianism, in the interest of animal rights. An older woman warned of contaminated water in our communities as she paced the interior of our circle: "There is mercury in our water." But as the day wore on, we heard no more of animal rights or contaminated water, and thus the global dimension of Giddens's definition of life politics was conspicuously absent.

We did hear about women's personal struggles with their health, their careers, and their lovers. Some women asked for help from the group. One who entered the center of the circle identified herself as a single mother. As she paced, she shared her frustration over a culture that does not value the labor of raising children. Her voice cracking, she asked the women present to affirm her. In response, women shouted out such affirmations as: "We value you." "You are doing noble work." "You are worthy." "Thank you for doing the most important work there is."

I was struck by this scene, by what was said and what was left unsaid, knowing that the devaluation of single mothering, indeed of all mothering, is expressed through material realities such as inadequate child care, public and private spaces unwelcoming to parents with their children, and the structure of work that forces an artificial divide between the personal the professional, I pondered the limits of the strategy of self-affirmation.[35] Was shoring up this mother's self-worth sufficient to ameliorate her suffering? I suspect she did not think so when she picked up her children from the sitter later that night, the warmth of support fading as the material realities closed in.

I am not suggesting we do away with spoken affirmations, but I ponder how the focus on an individual's need for validation inadvertently obscures the structural conditions that render single mothering, in this case, so difficult. Raising children without the support of a partner is a trial not simply because individual women do not hear often enough that they are worthy (although they most definitely do not). Single mothering is difficult because our society is structured as if all children are raised in nuclear heterosexual families with a (generous) wage-earning father and stay-at-home mother. To ease the burdens placed on single mothers would take radicalization of the world of work and the redistribution of resources, at least minimally. But this larger view of the problem did not appear to be foremost on the minds of the women I met at the Belly and Womb Conference. No doubt, they would agree that our personal problems are not ours alone and that solutions must come in the form of sweeping structural changes, as well as affirmations. But in that room, it was clear that the day's focus was *personal* transformation. The day, for those present, was about making internal change through the use of mystery, magic, and ritual and the gathering of comforting words—sister to sister.

Starkweather, at least, has grander hopes. At one point during the Women's Council, she appealed to the women present to rise up against social injustice. Her words punctuated by pounding on the drum she held between her legs, she intoned: "I want a small army of women. If we find our power, we can speak out and make change in the world." This call to action is the discourse of life politics, as discussed earlier, a form of social change that *begins* at the microlevel. But my sense was that social change was not what motivated most of the women in attendance. Rather, "revolution from within," to borrow the title from Gloria Steinem's book on self-esteem, constituted the day's agenda.[36]

This problem has plagued the U.S. women's movement at least since the heady early days of the second wave, when consciousness-raising (CR) groups emerged as a tactic of social change. Today, events like the Women's Council bear their legacy. CR groups attracted large numbers of American women to meetings in which they informally shared the injustices they noted in their day-to-day personal lives and linked those same injustices to the structural oppression of women. As Lisa Maria Hogeland observes, the relationship between CR and making social change was pragmatic: CR was "a starting point for feminism, a place from which to begin doing more public, activist organizing, rather than an end in itself or an investigative model."[37] That is, CR was seen as the initial step in identifying and actively resisting structural injustice, but it was not practiced without controversy, especially in the beginning.

In 1969 Dottie Zellner, a staff member of the Southern Conference Educational Fund (SCEF), wrote and circulated a memo that damned CR as "just therapy" and questioned whether the new independent women's liberation movement was really "political." In response, fellow staffer Carol Hanisch penned her own memo and sent it to the women's caucus of SCEF. Hanisch was an adherent of what came to be known as the "pro-woman line," a faction of the women's liberation movement that rejected "a spiritual, psychological, metaphysical or pseudo-historical explanation for women's oppression with a real, materialist analysis for why women do what we do." As Hanisch famously put it in her memo: "Women are messed over, not messed up!" She went on to defend CR as a form of political action and to stipulate her reasons for participating:

One of the first things we discover in these groups is that personal problems are political problems. There are no personal solutions at this time. There is only collective action for a collective solution. I went, and I continue to go, to these meetings because I have gotten a political understanding which all my reading, all my "political discussions," all my "political action," all my four-odd years in the movement never gave me. I've been forced to take off the rose-colored glasses and face the awful truth about how grim my life really is as a woman. I am getting a gut understanding of everything as opposed to the esoteric, intellectual understandings and noblesse oblige feelings I had in "other people's" struggles. [38]

A year later Shulamith Firestone and Anne Koedt edited the memo, attached to it a title now turned iconic phrase, "The Personal Is Political," and published it in their anthology *Notes from the Second Year*.[39] But in the case of feminist-spiritualist menstrual activism, in places like the Women's Council, the "political" of the equation drops out. Life politics gives way to self-transformation for self-transformation's sake.

What's the harm in that? The answer may depend on who you are.

UNDER THE RED TENT

Because of my interest in the feminist-spiritualist approach to menstruation, at the Belly and Womb Conference I attended two workshops but spent much of my time in the Red Tent, visiting the space at various points throughout the day. The first workshop I attended, "The Blood Mysteries: A Ritual of Empowerment for Maidens, Mothers, and Crones," was led by Opeyemi Parham, an allopathic family physician turned holistic healer (she playfully refers to herself as a "witch doctor") who was also, notably, one of the few menstrual activists of color in attendance. As Parham pulled back the heavy curtained "door" to the Red Tent, she whispered in each woman's ear, "The first blood mystery: women bleed, but they do not die." Once we were all seated, Parham led us through a series of guided visualizations to present a "cross-cultural perspective" that offered women "the idea that our bodies are sacred and that our blood and cycles are magical and potent."[40] Through these visualizations and the debriefing that followed, Parham presented an alternative framing of the menstrual cycle across the lifespan that departed from the ho-hum attitude or outright hostility that most contemporary western women adopt in relation to their menstrual cycles. She encouraged us to reflect deeply on our attitudes toward menstruation as young girls and young women, and toward menopause as middle-aged and older women, gently urging us to claim these life processes as sources of knowledge and power.

The Red Tent was also the site of another menstrually themed workshop, Sheri Winston's "Red Power—Honoring the Medicine Wheel of the Moon time: A Celebration of Menstrual Health, Tradition, and Wisdom." Winston's approach was more lighthearted and playful than Parham's, but I observed something fascinating, and even distressing, that morning. After the women settled, each woman menstruating at the time was offered a bindi (Winston was already wearing a bright red one on her forehead). I was struck by how easily she offered this Hindu symbol to a group of white women, none of whom, I guessed, identified as Hindu. No explanation of the history or original purpose of bindis was offered; in this context they were simply a decorative item that signified the menstruators among us. Bindis were abundant at the Belly and Womb Conference. Indeed, they are common at many feminist-spiritualist gatherings, although the rationale for wearing them was never, in my presence, articulated (I assume the bindi is taken to be symbolic of fertility). But what are the ramifications of groups of mostly white, western women appropriating a Hindu religious symbol, even one that is increasingly a fashionable accessory among Indians and other South Asians?

As Meenaskshi Gigi Durham points out, bindis (and other symbols of South Asian femininity, such as mehndi and nose rings) are now "ethnic chic."[41] Pop icons Madonna and Gwen Stefani have worn bindis, despite some South Asians finding this practice offensive, among them a South Asian Yale student, Sunita Puri: "Assigning new cultural meanings to symbols with very old traditions or deep personal significance is inappropriate and insensitive. It reduces the complexities of South Asian culture to mere physical items, rather than the continual process that culture is."[42]

Durham pursues her analysis of the cultural appropriation of symbols of South Asian femininity in the contexts of fashion and popular culture and asserts that the practice must be seen in terms of commodification.[43] Further, she argues, western appropriation of culturally specific symbols reifies historic and contemporary power differentials between the sexualized white woman and the disembodied Indian woman: "As long as White women are given the privilege of conferring meaning on these symbols, [Asian] and Asian American women's relationships to these symbols are undermined." Especially applicable to the feminist-spiritualist use of the bindi, Durham's explanation reveals the global dimensions of what might seem an isolated and localized practice: "An important aspect of this commodification is its western power base and the East-West relations at play: The recognition that western countries control the means of media production and marketing must accompany analysis of fashion and its entailments. Within this framework, the cultural appropriation of Eastern cultures as trends, styles, or exotic sexual displays can be understood in terms of issues of imperialism and dominance."[44]

Even more prevalent among feminist-spiritualists are the use of Native American drums and rattles, references to Native American practices such as the moon lodge, and oversimplified or romanticized belief systems attributed to Native American cultures, such as positive attitudes toward menstruation as a sacred time in which women are at their highest power. When I asked menstrual activists to "tell me when you first became interested in menstrual activism," the response from a feminist-spiritualist menstrual activist was representative: "I lived 'close to the land' for many years in the seventies and eighties and learned about many Native American ways, although I did not actively study them. When I heard about the moon-lodge practice of Native American women, it awakened me to the spiritual dimension of menstruation."[45] The level of this activist's engagement with "Native American ways" was not clear. Did she merely access information or did she participate in rituals of some kind, such as the moon lodge? Throughout my interviews, I heard similar stories that uncritically referenced and essentialized Native American practices and beliefs.

Cultural appropriation has met with swift criticism in other contexts. For example, when Toronto artist Andy Fabo deployed the symbolism of the sweat lodge in his work in the late 1980s, the public outcry led him to justify his choice. Of his explanation that a boyhood visit to the Museum of Plains Indians "had an incredible impact" on him, legal scholar Rosemary Coombe countered: "The sweat-lodge might indeed constitute a powerful symbolic image, but Fabo's use of it illustrated no reflexive consideration of the legacy of power that enabled him to exploit its symbolic excess." Absent such consideration, argues Coombe, the white artist's use of the sweat lodge reproduces the historic hierarchical relationship between the colonizer and the colonized.[46] In this formulation, the borrowing of a native practice is not harmless, even if the act is inspired by a sincere

appreciation. Coombe's point is that practices cannot be severed from their historical context—in this case, exploitation that made possible a white man's
access to the sacred life of indigenous North Americans subjected to genocide
and state repression.

But even harsh critics of appropriation do not begrudge individuals or groups
the right to learn about practices of cultures different from one's culture of origin.
Indeed, doing so can engender sensitivity and appreciation and may build cross-
cultural bridges. But if the activist who "did not actively study" Native American
ways adopted rituals ignorant of their meanings for their originators (at the very
least), this is problematic, although Durham acknowledges that the popularity of
appropriated symbols in youth culture may "speak to more than a desire to co-
opt the exotic." These practices can also be seen as "creative and complicated varieties of cultural hybridization, experimentation, and global-local intersections."[47]
Should white, western, feminist-spiritualist menstrual activists take the Red Tent
or moon lodge, the Hindu bindi, or even Middle Eastern dance (also a popular
feminist-spiritualist activity) out of their historical and cultural contexts? Is it
possible to use these symbols, rituals, and activities to endow their own rituals
with meaning without (albeit intentionally) reproducing raced power relations?

Is it possible to practice moon lodge or distribute bindis to menstruating
women in culturally sensitive ways? Maybe. Perhaps if the bindi is introduced
historically, referencing its original signification as a sacred Hindu symbol and
gradual evolution as a decorative accessory, the symbol would be seen in context.
Discussions could then follow regarding the implications of non-Indian and
non-Hindu women wearing the symbol. What is gained? What is potentially
lost? How might communities of mostly white, western women wearing bindis
appear to Indian and Hindu women? Does such a practice attract racially, ethnically, and religiously diverse women to menstrual activism or, more generally, to
feminist spirituality—or might it repel them? Until such conversations occur, I
fear that the use of culturally specific practices by Euro-Americans represents
women of color, by way of their traditions, as the exotic other.

Furthermore, given the overwhelming whiteness of the movement (or at least
the stark segregation that marks the movement, as I suggest in chapter 6), it
behooves the activists—if they hope to build a more ethnically, racially, and culturally diverse movement—to examine the ways cultural appropriation may
repel women who identify with cultures that have endured the injustices of white
and western imperialism and colonialism.[48] When activists uncritically and liberally appropriate cultural traditions, they practice a self-transformation that
may lack appeal to others. In this case, life politics becomes self-transformation
in the interest of the privileged. This may be another reason the feminist-
spiritualist movement endures yet remains on the fringe. The potential to
change a select number of individual lives is real and often realized, but, in the
final analysis, it leads largely to its own self-perpetuation.

Cultivating Body Literacy

While cross-cultural literacy was not evident in the discourse of the activists I encountered, literacy of another sort *was* prioritized—body literacy. Women use body literacy to develop self-awareness, that is, a working knowledge of how their bodies function, so that they can assess what is normal and what is not. In terms of reproductive and sexual health, women become body literate "when they can read and comprehend the signs, events and outcomes related to their menstrual cycles and are able to use this knowledge as a foundation for lifelong sexual and reproductive health choices."[49]

Several of the menstrual activists I met teach women how to chart their menstrual cycles, noting not only the days of their menstrual period, but also symptoms during the period and emotional and physiological changes throughout the month. Paying attention to one's body—discharge, headaches, cramps, energy level, sleep, exercise and diet patterns, and emotional states—can even reduce menstrual cycle disturbances. For example, in one controlled study, women who experienced menstrual cycle irregularities, including amenorrhea (no period), oligomenorrhea (infrequent or light menstruation), and regular anovulatory cycles (periods with no ovulation), found their cycles normalized after one year of consistent charting.[50] Some menstrual activists, including health educators trained in the Justisse Method for Fertility Management (whose centerpiece is menstrual cycle charting), claim that women who experience difficulty getting pregnant often conceive once they learn to chart.[51]

But before a woman can chart, she needs to learn the basics of the menstrual cycle. To explain, I return to Winston's workshop in the Red Tent. To illustrate the menstrual cycle, Winston drew a circle, divided it into phases, and linked the cycle of ovulation and menstruation to the cycles of birth, death, and rebirth, reminding participants of the link between menses, the moon, and the tides. During preovulation and ovulation, she said, women tend to be more energetic, social, and creative. When women bleed, Winston explained, "we turn our gaze completely inside and figure out what's not working" Next, she brought out a basket of alternative menstrual products and stated: "We have two choices: We can hold the blood in (and be more like men) or let it flow." At the conclusion of the workshop, one participant exclaimed, shaking her head: "Wow! The things they didn't tell you."

Winston has been teaching the link between menstrual cycle physiology and emotional states to promote body literacy for more than twenty years. At eighteen or nineteen, she began redefining her own relationship to her menstrual cycle, and like others I spoke to, she cited Native American practices and beliefs as inspiration. While practicing pagan and Native American ceremonies, Winston explained, she learned from native leaders that menstrual blood is powerful. Soon thereafter, she learned of Tamara Slayton's work and began using reusable sea sponges during her period; as a result, she "just had this very different relationship with [her] own bleeding from then on."[52] Winston's choice to switch to sea sponges marks a transformation in her consciousness, and thus her willingness to interact authentically with her body and its processes. When a menstruator uses sea sponges, a reusable alternative to single-use tampons, she must wash out the sponge after each use. This practice requires coming into direct contact with one's menses, a kind of body-consciousness interaction that is rare in today's disposable, menstruation-averse culture.

Today, Winston, a midwife and women's healthcare provider by training, offers more than thirty different workshops on sexuality and women's health. Through her teaching, she has an opportunity to encourage women to similarly redefine their connection, not only with their bleeding, but also more generally with their bodies. Bodily fluids (particularly those associated with reproduction) can be wonderful and wondrous, neutral, or disgusting, claims Winston. In a culture that constructs women's bodies, to use philosopher Elizabeth Grosz's term, as "volatile," or as unpredictable entities that must be controlled and contained, it is not uncommon for a woman to find her blood repulsive. In this case, finds Winston, it is "too late" to reverse the alienation from her body. "It starts with first blood," she claims.[53] A woman's response to breastfeeding is also significant, says Winston, because it is forged in her relationship with her menses. Psychologist Ros Bramwell supports this claim, having explored the socially constructed link between menstrual blood and breast milk in western societies: "If women internalise views that their bodies are disgusting, that they need to buy products to be 'liberated' from the constraints of their biology, that their bodies can be defined in terms of their capacity to provide male sexual pleasure, such views will form an important component of their attitude to breastfeeding."[54]

Yet the emphasis through workshops such as Winston's and Opeyemi Parham's is on the individual woman and her personal relationship with her body, not the disembodied culture of consumption that reinforces the mind-body split. Again, the focus is on the self: my body, my period, my health. ALisa Starkweather's wish to recruit a "small army of women" to fight for social justice is lost in the Red Tent, where women participate in *self*-transformation, not social transformation.

Similarly, Kami McBride's "Women's Wisdom" workshop series seeks to strip away the baggage and bias that shape dominant understandings of the menstrual cycle and to inspire a different personal awareness about menstruation. She hopes that women will emerge from her workshops both body literate and energized social agitators. Recently, she has been recruiting young women into future workshops. A few months after completing "Women's Wisdom," I received a written appeal to underwrite the workshop fee for interested young women who would otherwise not be able to attend. McBride's aim is to get information into the hands and minds of young women (including those of limited means) sooner rather than

later. Former workshop attendees testify to this need. As one former student
wrote, "Every woman should have access to this rich, wonderful information. I
wish I had been able to take this course as a teenager."[55] Body literacy in this view
ideally begins in youth and develops throughout the lifetime.

For the three-part workshop series I attended, nineteen women caravanned
to McBride's rural northern California home and herb school (I attended the
first and third workshops). We entered her modest wood-hewn building to the
Celtic strains of Loreena McKennitt. Some women knew one another from
McBride's other well-established series centered on herb lore and use. Others
were local or nearly local (San Francisco was only one hour's drive west), and
others were connected to feminist spirituality or natural health care in some way.
McBride began the day with a critique of the "crash-course approach to the
female cycles of life, which leave us open to medical experimentation, accidents,
et cetera." She asked if we felt prepared for our own cycles; no one answered yes.
McBride connected this common lack of preparedness with sexual abuse and
eating disorders, associating early detachment from the body with later problems (I privately connected it with the memory of an entire roomful of women
at the Belly and Womb Conference, each admitting that she struggled with her
body). "When we disregard our bodies, we disregard ourselves and our power,"
McBride told us. As she talked, the workshop participants nodded in agreement.
In side conversations, they spoke of other risks associated with detachment from
our bodies—breast cancer, allergies, alcohol and other drug abuse, and domestic violence.

Our day was both didactic and interactive. McBride helped us "get in touch
with our bodies" at multiple levels: intellectual, physical, emotional, and visceral.
The body-literate woman, her workshop curriculum implied, integrates varied
forms of knowledge. We broke into small groups and told stories of our first
menstruation, ostensibly to reclaim a lost history that can contribute to self-
awareness. (Mine: The winter of my eighth-grade year, I discovered a brown stain
and went ice skating with friends afterward, feeling older, wiser, a bit special. I
wanted that period to keep up with my friends,' but my appreciation for my
period quickly gave way to annoyance, shame, and even dread.) We danced. We
made art. We role-played. We honored the menstruating women among us, who
were invited to wear a bindi to mark their menstrual status (with no accompanying
discussion of bindis). We shared our lunch in a sumptuous healthful potluck.

McBride's focus was clearly the health and well-being of individual women,
but she hastened to remind us to think beyond the self. While sharing her belief
that "this experience is for you," she suggested we "use [it] to end the wars." I
was struck by this statement of life politics, because, as I've discussed, feminist-
spiritualist discourse typically does not explicitly connect the development of
menstrual pride to body literacy as a step toward social change. But even when
this link *is* made, concrete follow-through is lacking.

Body literacy, through discussions and group sharing, carries great potential as cultural resistance. Imagine the power of legions of informed, self-reliant women who feel empowered enough to rely less on institutionalized health care and more on their own resourcefulness! When such women seek help, they are prepared to articulately advocate for their needs. As I pointed out in chapter 3, when earlier feminist health activists founded organizations and published self-help guides, they imagined precisely this outcome. Believing that only lack of information stood between women and their potential for self-care, activists worked to connect women with the resources for developing healthy self-awareness. In a telling continuity with its recent past, today's menstrual activists are still at it. But is it enough?

Body literacy is part of a more general quest for the self-transformation that some activists hope will lead to change on a grander scale. Some, like McBride and Starkweather, do not see it as end in itself, at least not in the abstract. However, their suggestion that individual women transform their renovated consciousness into measurable action appears to lack currency with the women who seek out their workshops and conferences. And because they fail to help women make the link between *their* personal and *our* collective need to organize for social change, self-transformation is the single end result. The women come for personal reasons: to learn how *their* menstrual cycles work, to heal *their* ailing bodies, and to reckon with *their* painful histories while ignoring the equally painful histories of others.

There is a sense of separation at work here, not to mention a subtle ethnocentrism. Mine. Yours. Ours. Theirs. Self. Other. *My* self-transformation. *My* body literacy. And when it feels good, traditions of *their* culture can be deployed in the service of *our* self-improvement. To demarcate and sustain these separations, race and class privileges are invoked, though often not consciously. Indeed, unspoken privilege is the engine that propels feminist-spiritualist menstrual activism. The project of self-improvement, after all, is itself a privilege and one that takes cultural capital to enact.

Privilege and Accessibility

Because of the ubiquitous strength of the menstrual taboo, activists meet a range of negative reactions from apathy to outrage when they articulate a menstruation-positive perspective. Thus, the burden is on the menstrual activists to present this unfamiliar information in ways that attract rather than repel. But there appears to be little effort to draw in women who do not hold the perspective of white, middle-class, college-educated, feminist-identified women. That is, the privilege of the activists, unintentionally it seems, constructs menstrual activism as inaccessible for many women.[56] The materials used to spread awareness make their pitch to women already steeped in a New Age, women-centered sensibility

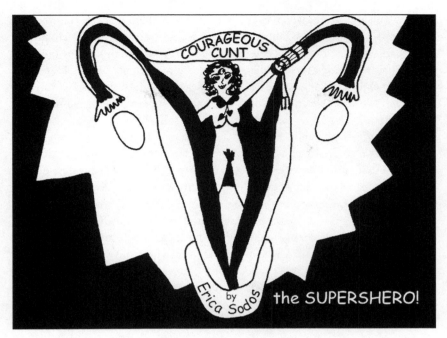

Figure 4. Erica Sodos, "Courageous Cunt," *Moonflow* magazine, 2005. Courtesy of the artist.

infused with spiritualist meaning. For example, feminist-spiritualist alternative menstrual discourse is rife with words like "magic," "mystery," "power," "sacred," "gifts," and "healing"; book covers typically feature moons, dragons, flowers in bloom, and goddesses. These words and images function as signals or codes to a particular community whose members share a worldview.

Sometimes a well-meaning activist overstates the power of menstruation to transform women's lives, as happens in Erica Sodos's periodical *Moonflow*, a modest, small-circulation magazine that published eight issues (or "cycles," as the masthead stated) before shutting down. Carrying the tagline "dedicated to a woman's monthly cycle" and printed in black and white, the 4 × 6 magazine numbered thirty-one pages of features and regular segments, such as a Q&A piece titled "Dear Moon Time Mama" and a Flow Tracking Moon Calendar (again, in the interest of promoting body literacy). *Moonflow* typically concluded with the editor and publisher's hand-drawn comic strip "Courageous Cunt."

Although playful and merely symbolic, this strip likely alienates the very population it aspires to support. We encounter a woman with toddlers at her feet, lamenting: "How am I going to take care of my babies? I don't have *any money*!" Next, we see Courageous Cunt, arms spread wide and cape flowing, announcing: "This is not right! These sisters believe that they are poor. I must help them see the powerful abundance which lives inside of each of them." The next frame features the mother street peddling. Courageous Cunt activates her "ferociously flowing forward cycle" (which ostensibly dispenses "sacred moontime blood"). In the final two frames, the penniless mother is shown on the phone accepting a job—with child care included! The panhandler sits beneath the blazing sun and enthuses: "Wow! It's a miracle! Now I have enough money to return home to my great satisfying job and wonderful family." It is unlikely, given the typical audience for feminist-spiritualist menstrual activism, that many poor women would encounter this comic strip, but I can imagine the response it would elicit from them. The suggestion that the way out of poverty is through a heavy dose of self-esteem smacks of the "lift yourself up by your bootstraps" discourse of those who fail to see the workings of structural inequality and the myth of meritocracy.

The written word is a potent if not dangerous tool for feminist-spiritualist menstrual activists. The dissemination of knowledge helps to cultivate a sense of "we" that binds them, even if they have never met. A rash of books published between 1994 and 2005 combine reinterpretations of menstrual taboos with "how-to" guides to honor, reclaim, and celebrate menstruation. Important to movement vitality, these books encourage the circulation of alternative attitudes and model the unconventional approaches at the heart of feminist-spiritualist menstrual activism. Diffuse and largely decentralized, the movement relies on the production and exchange of information as a means to establish collective identity.

My bookshelves bulge with titles, all introduced to me by feminist-spiritualist menstrual activists, that reframe menstruation as a sacred, powerful, and creative time for *all* women. Not surprisingly, the texts teeter on the edge of popular literature. I found most of them through used booksellers or in New Age bookshops. Among the feminist-spiritualists, however, they are well known and often cross-referenced. Though each is unique, they share a spiritualist orientation (leaving the biophysiology to scientists and health-care providers) and essentialist conceptions of womanhood. Their aim is self-empowerment, not social change, although some authors nod to the transformative power of legions of strong, healthy, self-aware women. The presence of social analysis is uneven, typically occurring only at the beginning of a text in the form of an explanation of menstruation's second-class social status. A passage from *Red Moon: Understanding and Using the Gifts of the Menstrual Cycle* is representative: "For centuries, the woman's menstrual cycle has been viewed with something approaching revulsion and contempt; it was seen as dirty, a sign of sin and its existence reinforced women's inferior position in male dominated society. Menstruation is still viewed today as a biological disadvantage to women, making them emotional, unreasoning and unreliable workers."[57]

Books containing similar sentiments range from self-published practical guides, such as Kami McBride's *105 Ways to Celebrate Menstruation* (e.g., "wear a red bindi on your forehead," "sing a song to the moon"), to larger-circulation trade texts.[58] During my fieldwork studying feminist-spiritualist menstrual activism, titles I heard referenced include: *New Moon Rising: Reclaiming the Sacred Rites of Menstruation* (infused with "Native American spirituality"); *Dragon Time: Magic and Mystery of Menstruation; Moon Days: Creative Writings about Menstruation; The Wild Genie: The Healing Power of Menstruation; The Seven Sacred Rites of Menarche; Women's Rites of Passage: Reconnecting to the Source of Feminine Power* (with companion CD), the previously cited *Red Moon: Understanding and Using the Gifts of the Menstrual Cycle*; and *A Time to Celebrate: A Celebration of a Girl's First Menstrual Period*. Some books, like the oft-referenced *Wise Wound: Myths, Realities, and Meanings of Menstruation*, explore the social meanings of ancient taboos, endeavoring to reinterpret them, much as do *Red Flower: Rethinking Menstruation* and Slayton's *Reclaiming the Menstrual Matrix*. Poet Judy Grahn's alternative historical account of menstrual rites, *Blood, Bread and Roses: How Menstruation Created the World*, engages mythology and anthropology to boldly (and at times, shakily) assert that women's seclusion during menstruation shaped mathematics, cosmetics, astronomy, and cooking, as well as marriage and mourning customs. The afore-mentioned *Blood Magic*, edited by Buckley and Gottlieb, offers cross-cultural comparative analyses that challenge the universality of the menstrual taboo. Menstrual activists often cite Grahn's and Buckley and Gottlieb's books to legit-imize their work as rooted in history and anthropology.[59]

Lara Owen's *Her Blood Is Gold: Celebrating the Power of Menstruation*, a book that draws on myth, tradition, and personal stories, was among the most often cited by the feminist-spiritualists I interviewed (and among the websites and books I analyzed). The author opens with her own journey into her "menstrual mysteries," which involved purging her life of nearly all material goods, quitting her job, and moving to another country. Through a series of experiences and introspections, Owen was led to recognize "the value and pleasure of [her] peri-ods [as] an opening . . . into a deep appreciation of being a woman," but she does not acknowledge the constellation of privileges that led her to this appreciation.[60]

Would it be sufficient if she did acknowledge the relationship between her social location and her life choices? I am not sure, but at least such an acknowl-edgment would challenge the assumption that any woman can reclaim menstru-ation and find spiritual fulfillment and that doing so is simply a matter of will. When privilege is named, institutional forces that make actions such as relocation, choosing unemployment, and having ample time for self-reflection a reality are brought into focus.

The point is that, through the lens of feminist-spiritualism, the means to reframe menstruation and empower women to embrace rather than reject this embodied process is left to the individualized practices of women with privilege. For example, in the introduction to *The Wild Genie: The Healing Power of Menstruation*, author Alexandra Pope explains the purpose of her book: "*The*

Wild Genie is a self care guide for all women in their menstruating years who want to enjoy their cyclical nature and experience a long, fulfilling and healthy life—looking utterly gorgeous to the end!" Pope concludes *The Wild Genie* with recipes and instructions for addressing minor health problems related to menstruation, such as cramps and bloating, or for improving general wellness: various teas, miso soup, lemon water, and rejuvulac (a fermented drink made from wheat sprouts). Instructions for enjoying a "luxurious Epsom salt bath" and making your own castor oil (for premenstrual ailments) and linseed pack (for generalized discomforts) are included as well.[61]

While these recommendations may resonate for some women, particularly those with flexible schedules, a coparent and ample retreat space in their homes, and time and money to shop for supplies (many not readily available in conventional stores), they likely ring hollow for women with less privilege: those who work blue- or pink-collar jobs, exist on fixed incomes, and enjoy little privacy, and mothers with limited time (or inclination) and few resources to practice such self-care. Pope sometimes acknowledges the difficulty of women's taking time off to "practice moon lodge" (or even a modest adaptation). as well as accessing the journals, teas, and baths, but she urges women to make it work *somehow*.

The message is clear in Pope's text, as well as in others I studied: Menstruation is a special time in a woman's life and should be honored appropriately. Most suggestions for accomplishing this require interrupting work and other daily responsibilities. Within the sphere of feminist-spiritualist menstrual activism, the prescription to take time out to renew and rejuvenate is common. McBride's "Women's Wisdom" workshop encouraged participants to consciously honor the first day of menses, because the menstrual period is a time of drawing within and practicing self-reflection. If the menstruating woman interrupts her routine and rests, she is more likely to tap into her "menstrual wisdom." Similarly, under the Red Tent, Winston asked her workshop participants: "How can you honor that first day of bleeding? To honor that deep spiritual place?" She then offered how she does it: "I don't cook, clear, or serve anyone; I don't want to be bugged."

Hemitra Crecraft, developer of multimedia materials, ritualist and co-owner of Heart of the Goddess online boutique and self-described "New Paradigm Teacher/Celebrationist of Women's Cycles," has managed to carve out time and space to honor her menstrual period for many years. When I asked her when she first became interested in menstrual activism, she e-mailed me a list key life events, including encountering a Native American song: "May 1959—my menarche honoring dinner with my family—initiated by my father in response to my delight in becoming a woman; Summer 1971 Apache Girl Rite of Passage song at Museum of Natural History, NY (felt that I knew the song, even though I had never heard it before—yearned to complete this initiation); summer 1976 Moon Lodge initiation Switzerland; practiced moon lodge for 17 years (withdrew to bedroom and rested for one–three days every month when menstruating to renew myself)."[62] Crecraft's narrative is a compelling illustration of the centrality of privilege in the enactment of alternative menstrual practices. Such feminist-spiritualist menstrual activists enjoy their place among relatively privileged women but fail, I venture, to attract women who do not share their socioeconomic advantages. How do the feminist-spiritualists keep their wing of the menstrual activism movement alive?

COMMODIFYING SELF-TRANSFORMATION

Comedic performer and zinester Chella Quint told me "I find that when people react dubiously before they see our show because they think we might be 'hippy-dippy-moon-love-merchants,' there is a lot of mistrust—and I've always wondered if it was because they think we're going to sell them some kind of faux-spiritual shtick for huge amounts of cash."[63] The pursuit of self-transformation has become a niche market and some, like Quint, wish to distance themselves. When I asked each woman, "How would you describe yourself?" none identified herself as a business owner or entrepreneur, but twelve of the fourteen activists who fell into the subcategory feminist-spiritualist either sold products (books, CDs, kits, etc.) or offered various services for which they charged, such as rituals, workshops, and individual consultations. Activists, cognizant of ample numbers of privileged women eager to develop an alternative menstrual consciousness, have channeled their energies into the establishment of small women-owned and -operated businesses that meet this need. Reactions to this approach are mixed.

But let me be clear: I do not necessarily find fault with their founding these businesses; I certainly do not cast aspersions on some women's creative means of earning or supplementing their incomes. As a participant-observer at numerous events that charged a fee, I have seen firsthand the valuable impact workshops and conferences have on participants. And I do not doubt the sincerity of the organizers of these events; they genuinely aim to help women lead healthier, more fulfilling lives. Furthermore, I am quite certain that none of the small-business owners I encountered is getting rich off the proceeds they earn doing this work and selling their products. My point is not to judge the women who do their activism *through* commerce, but to suggest that this method of reaching individuals and making change is the means by which feminist-spiritualist menstrual activism has endured over the years yet remained marginal. If movement participants had not found a way to sustain themselves through their businesses, their activism likely would have faded away.

Described on her website as a leader in the Philadelphia Women's Spirituality community since the mid 1980s, Crecraft has worked independently and in collaboration with sister feminist-spiritualists. She and colleagues Sue King and Anne Strawbridge run Woman Wisdom, a small independent publishing company. During her career, Crecraft has designed multimedia programs, led various celebrations (her passion is girls' menarcheal coming-of-age celebrations), and codesigned numerous educational programs. Between 1990 and 2000, Crecraft was co-owner of the brick-and-mortar Heart of the Goddess boutique, described as "a women's spirituality center and sanctuary for women's healing, learning, celebration ... and sacred shopping."[64] The Heart of the Goddess reopened in 2004 as an online boutique.

I first met Crecraft at Starkweather's 2005 Belly and Womb Conference. As a "special surprise" for conference attendees, Crecraft held a screening of her rough-cut DVD "From Girl to Woman" (part of her Everyday Magic for Girls series, the DVD accompanies a girl's workbook and adult guidebook retailing at $48.95). I was intrigued by the DVD's multicultural presentation of menarcheal rituals and reframing of menstruation as a positive, affirming life experience in opposition to the hygienic crisis orientation in recent U.S. history documented by historian Joan Brumberg. For instance, the film referenced and depicted Hopi kachina dolls, Apache coming-of-age ceremonies, and the Japanese Coming of Age Day (January 14). Faces of many colors appear throughout the film (as do butterflies and flowers distinguished by their vulvar shapes).

In a room filled almost exclusively with white women, I struggled with the multicultural emphasis of the film. Genuine outreach or cultural appropriation? I wondered. Messages such as "You are part of a new community of women who celebrate their bodies and honor their moon time" suggested again the deployment of menstruation as a unifying experience for *all* women. This statement fails to acknowledge that diverse contexts produce diverse responses to menstruation. There is no unified community to which girls are welcomed upon their menarche. Indeed, there is no universal experience of menstruation.

Nevertheless, the point of Crecraft's film is clear: Menstruation is a gift that should be celebrated, and richly, perhaps by choosing from an extensive line of "goddess garb" available for those who wish to "sacredly shop" at "Heart of the Goddess: Your Source for Goddess Everything." In addition to a "Coming of Age: From Bud to Flower" multimedia kit, the boutique's website suggests a number of additional items for the celebration, including a menarche ceremonial dress, Goddess of Celebration necklace, Spirit Healer pendant, Nile River Goddess Drum, Butterfly Suncatcher, Purple Fairy Journal, Spiral Goddess statue, and menarche party favors (such as Pocket Magic Dust) and decorations (such as ceremonial banners). It is easy, in this case, to lose sight of the activism among the inventory.

A smaller-scale celebration kit is available from entrepreneurial mother-daughter pair Ann Short and Helynna Brooke, the latter a cofounder of the Red Web Foundation. In 1998 they developed a First Moon kit to assist in what they believed was the proper ritual celebration of menarcheal girls. In the period of time after a ritual they designed for Brooke's own daughter and niece, they decided to establish a web-based mail-order business, making it possible for more and more families to mark first menstruation in a positive way. On their website, Short and Brooke assert: "Womanhood needs to be defined by women. For too long it has been defined by men, the media and advertisements. If we do not help girls define womanhood, they will be defined. Older women who matter to the girl should be a part of teaching the skills to survive successfully and conscientiously in our culture as women."[65] For twenty-eight dollars plus shipping and handling, one receives a tidy white box containing a few modest materials—customizable invitations, ceremonial candles, cloth, and a "speaking stone" in a velvet pouch. One can make a bow of the included hot-pink ribbon to transform the shipping box into a keepsake box. Additionally, the kit contains a script on audiocassette (and accompanying transcript booklet) to shape the coming-of-age ritual, intended for the girl-turned-woman and the women in her immediate community—mother, grandmothers, aunts, and other women special to the guest of honor.

Innovative materials such as those created by Crecraft and by Brooke and Short may indeed be helpful to those who wish to create a more positive menstrual experience for girls. Recognizing that menstrual shame and alienation from the body are the consequences of androcentric western constructions of embodiment, menstruation-affirming actions may usher in the empowered body awareness that (ideally) promises to inoculate young women against perniciously gendered discrimination.

Nevertheless, I take issue with the focus of these materials and more generally with the menstrual activist discourse of coming of age that marks menarche as a girl's definitive maturation from girl to woman. I am troubled by the feminist-spiritualist tendency to collapse womanhood with reproduction and the conspicuous absence of girls as agents of their own menstrual experience. Crecraft's film, for example, links fertility to womanhood in narration such as, "You are like a butterfly magically changing from girl to woman." Accompanying footage of a menarcheal celebration, the honoree dressed in white, a wreath of flowers circling her blond head, is another of ALisa Starkweather's chants:

Red Bud Blossoming
You are Opening
Bleeding is Flowering
A New Woman Walks on the Earth.[66]

The feminized trope of the (predictably red) rosebud—tight, protected, innocent, and untouched—represents the premenarcheal girl who, once she begins to bleed, becomes open, accessible, exposed. The physiological readiness or near readiness for sexual reproduction (many girls are anovulatory for the first several menstrual cycles) signals her transition to womanhood. Now she claims the identity "woman." No other single development marks this transition with such poignancy or incontrovertible "evidence" of new womanhood. First Moon's

"Instructions for the Young Woman" begins: "Your mother has suggested that you be the center of attention in a ceremony celebrating your menarche and *entry into womanhood*."[67] I ask, What are the hazards of equating menstruation (the beginning of female fertility) with maturation to womanhood? Biologically, of course, menarche does indicate that the female body is ready (or nearly ready) to reproduce. However, defining menstruation as the "gateway to womanhood" (as Crecraft does in the script of her film) reinscribes a reproductive paradigm that conflates "womanhood" and "reproductive being." Is the essential feminine thus reduced to future mother? And if so, how does this paradigm limit girls' and women's sense of their multiplicity and self-determination to shape their own lives? This reductive causal logic ignores the role of intellectual and emotional maturity, important variables in this developmental equation. Ironically, this discourse tends to reify the mind/body dualism, a value-laden bifurcation that prioritizes that which is male over that which is female—the very hierarchization that feminist-spiritualists oppose in their embrace of cultural feminism.[68] After all, the girl who begins menstruating at age nine or ten is rarely considered a woman; she is a child who has started her period. Of course, the discourse of menarche equals womanhood is not particular to the feminist-spiritualists. Many girls who announce (or more likely, whisper) that they are having their first period have heard someone exclaim, "Now you are a woman." But when feminist-spiritualists actively ritualize this transition and call discursive and symbolic attention to fertility as the mark of maturity, their message amplifies the valorization of reproduction in women's lives.

Another problem: Do girls want menarcheal celebrations? If so, do they want spiritually infused celebrations in which they, the maidens, are anointed by a group of older women in flowing gowns? During extended interviews with eleven girls, Elizabeth Kissling described Hemitra Crecraft's "Coming of Age." The girls' reactions (with one exception) were uniformly negative, ranging from nonplussed to repulsed, for example: "I wouldn't want to celebrate something that's not very exciting, you know?" and "No way! I wouldn't do that. I'd say, 'Skip it, Mom!'"[69] Such reactions make one wonder whom these rituals are for. Some critics suggest that menarcheal rituals are designed by women who are dealing with their late-onset loss surrounding their own menarche (I didn't have a ceremony; no one honored me; I was made to feel ashamed about my body— but it is going to be different for my daughter.) Not coincidentally, some third-wave feminists are the first to question such rituals. Do we, as spoken-word slam poet (and minor third-wave celebrity) Alix Olson asks, *hide* behind our daughters? In "Daughter," she fantasizes about the unshackled, rabble-rousing life her someday–girl child will lead. Then she muses:

and it's funny how we hide behind these Daughters
hide ahead of our own Herstories

scared of ourselves
scared of the world
scared of Someone
who made us
one way
or another.[70]

Jennifer Baumgardner and Amy Richards in their 2000 third-wave feminist call-to-arms, *Manifesta*, critique the then-nascent "girl power movement" by hypothesizing that the engineers of many so-called girls' empowerment activities are feminist women seeking to redress their own injustices through their daughters, both figurative and literal. Olson and Baumgardner and Richards prod adult women to get busy working on their own issues and leave the girls alone. I must admit it is hard not to hear second- versus third-wave feminist tensions playing out in this defense of girls, especially when the objections devolve into an uncritical view of menstruation. Here we are, talking past each other again. Many girls, suggest Baumgardner and Richards, would not find menarcheal rituals empowering, because periods aren't much to celebrate. In this reinforcement of the menstrual status quo, they write that "as two women who just hit thirty and who are facing at least two more decades of generously supporting Tambrands and some ibuprofen company, we don't think we need to say too much about why girls complain about their monthly blood rite."[71] There is no doubt that most girls are predisposed to think negatively about their periods; after all, they are reading from the cultural script. When my daughter, aged twelve, told me that she expected to hate her period because "everybody says it's awful," my heart sank. (You can imagine the kinds of fantasies I had entertained about how my daughter's first menstruation would be different.) But Baumgardner and Richards seem unable or unwilling to acknowledge the socially constructed reality of negative attitudes toward menstruation. Girls may dread their periods, but must they? ask feminist-spiritualists like the creators of First Moon kits.

Perhaps something—or someone—is missing in such kits. In *Manifesta*, Baumgardner and Richards describe First Moon with contempt, noting the absence of girls themselves as cocreators of the ritual. From the feminist-spiritualist perspective, girls are to be celebrated—that is, to be acted upon—by a well-meaning community that likely includes individuals nostalgic for their own missed opportunity years ago. I agree that girls as agents are conspicuously missing from the discourse of feminist spiritualism. In Crecraft's film, for example, a visual feast of still images of girls engaged in ritual, girls laughing, girls looking contemplative, and so on, we hear the voice of only one girl who enthusiastically explains why she chooses to honor, not dread, her period. The inclusion of her narrative is powerful, but its singularity ultimately calls attention to the namelessness and voicelessness of every other girl we see. Crecraft's soothing middle-aged voiceover carries the message. I am left wondering (fully aware of the irony), What *do* girls want?

Coming-of-age rituals are intended to initiate girls into womanhood beyond the usual de facto rituals—first sexual encounter, first cigarette, first time driving a car—but are they in the best interest of girls (eventually) becoming women? Do girls want this recognition, even if we believe that in an ideal world they should? When I listened to the First Moon audiocassette, which introduces, justifies, and details the ceremony, I wondered how the mother's and grandmother's voices and words, those of a middle-aged woman and her mother, would resonate for girls who, at the age of first menstruation, are unlikely to feel celebratory. Given the near impenetrability of the dominant cultural narrative of menstruation, it is incumbent upon entrepreneur activists like Short, Brooke, and Crecraft to meet girls where they are if they hope to transform such deeply entrenched attitudes.

But if I listen to the activists with my maternal ear, I am somewhat comforted and affirmed. It is easy to imagine that there are other mothers like me who want to counter the hegemony of the negative menstrual mindset but don't know where to begin. I am not alone. A Google search of the terms "menstruation" and "ritual" produces 189,000 hits. There is a market for products related to these experiences. The question is, Who's buying them? The feminist-spiritualist menstrual activists may find their most receptive audience among mothers. In the language of the marketplace, they are the consumers; they hold the checkbooks.

Whether these well-meaning mothers serve their daughters' needs remains an open question. I offer a personal anecdote that illustrates the gulf between mothers' and daughters' needs. In spite of my (rehearsed) nonchalant overtures, when my daughter had her first period, she wasn't interested in a ritual, party, or celebration of any kind—no menarcheal gown or Pocket Magic Dust for her. Her stepdad and I were able to convince her to dine with just her immediate family at a local Mexican restaurant. At her request, the reason for the special dinner was never mentioned at the table.

Though clearly not for everyone, materials like those developed by Brooke and Short and Crecraft do facilitate an alternative experience of menarche that resonates for some young women and their families. First Moon has been in business since 1996. Crecraft has been developing and marketing new products since 1980. Starkweather's events, of which the Belly and Womb Conference is only one, are popular and well attended year after year. McBride's workshops fill up rapidly, too; I nearly did not get my own registration in before she ran out of space.[72] These events and products are a part of a vibrant niche market that is not yet saturated. But can the ceremonies be separated from the consumerist impulse? Does ritual require commercially produced props? Given the large number of books, workshops, periodicals, conferences, consultations, and products for sale, it is sometimes hard to separate the activism from the business side of challenging the menstrual status quo.

But maybe a more generous interpretation is possible. Perhaps, as I've suggested, the business of menstrual activism has become the lifeblood of the movement. Without it, activists might burn out or fade away as the demands of jobs and families sap their energy. Making feminist-inspired social change a commodity may raise the ire of many, but in spite of the so-called cheesy approach to feminism, feminist spiritualism has endured for thirty years. The feminist-spiritualists have survived—some would say outlived—the second wave to witness the emergence of the newest expression of the menstrual activism movement, the radical menstruation wing. The feminist-spiritualist message, in the hyperconsumerist U.S. culture, may proliferate more readily through the means of moving product. A trade book may reach many more people than a volunteer-run workshop offered seasonally. Through consumerism, menstrual activists at once profit and make heard their agenda of a profound cultural shift that celebrates (rather than denigrates) menstruation. But while the activist messages are radical, the means are accommodationist; feminist-spiritualists graft themselves to the capitalist machinery in a bid for currency and survival while working at the level of the individual. I appreciate the minefield I have walked into. Some find this analysis overly sympathetic, among them Elizabeth Kissling, author of *Capitalizing on the Curse*, who challenged me to pump up my critique of what she called "a shopping for social change vibe that contributes to [menstrual activism's] ineffectiveness" and pointed out that it takes not only privilege and cultural capital to participate in this wing of the movement, but also capital in the literal sense.[73]

At the same time, consider the exchange I had with a key figure among the feminist-spiritualists, ALisa Starkweather, who suggested I include in this book a list of activist resources to enable readers to connect with those I encountered during my fieldwork. Starkweather was dissatisfied with the result, a list of currently active initiatives limited to those that did not sell products or services. In an e-mail, she asked: "I wonder why keep this information too from women? What do you fear in giving women avenues, resources and brave women who are pioneering to bring us a new future? Why shut the doors?" When I outlined my critique of feminist spiritualism's merchandising, Starkweather hastened to point out that she mounts her events without assets, college degree, formal training of any kind, or staff to assist her, adding: "Oh yes I know what is sacred, particularly from the feminine, can be bought, sold and used beyond our comprehension. But my own intentions need to be aligned with this if I am simply going down as a profit-based business on spiritual feminism. It makes me laugh and cry."[74]

While I do not intend to write off any of the activists as merely profit-seeking individuals, I maintain that a services/products-for-fee model of activism is limiting. Even if I set aside the consumerist impulse in this wing of the movement for a moment, feminist-spiritualist menstrual activism's embrace of an "I bleed therefore I am" brand of cultural feminism is problematic. Furthermore, tactics that cater to women of privilege on a self-centered quest for transformation represent a compromised strategy for social change. A more careful reckoning of the appropriation of culture, the politics of privilege, and an essentialist conception of womanhood must be addressed before feminist spiritualism can swing the doors wide open. Feminist-spiritualist menstrual activism may succeed in transforming individual lives among a small cadre of women, but it fails to unite individual change with collective action. The life politics of feminist-spiritualist menstrual activism is partial. While the movement endures, it remains a mystical, magical world that appeals to few and touches fewer.

CHAPTER 5

Radical Menstruation

Women's bodies are different,
what a perfect market,
tell them that they're dirty,
we will make them smell like roses.
I'm gonna take care of myself—your fucking greed makes
    me choke. Aisles and aisles of pretty boxes
to make us odorless, hairless, tasteless,
make us just the way they want us,
but their products will fucking kill us.
                    —The Haggard, "Tampons," *A Bike City Called Greasy*

Yonah EtShalom was an early bloomer. At age sixteen she attended a Bloodsisters workshop at a local anarchist community center, where she heard talk of menstruation laced with good doses of humor, including:

Question: How do you know if a squatter is menstruating?
Answer: She's only got one sock on.

EtShalom admits that she had to find out that a squatter is someone who occupies a house they do not own (a practice often linked with punk subculture) before she could make the connection. The joke was a play on the punk do-it-yourself ethic, or DIY, a commitment to self-reliance that thumbs its nose at commercialization and hyperconsumption, including, as this joke implies, care of the menstruating body. Many punks don't buy menstrual supplies, especially name-brand products made by multinational corporations. Rather, when and where they can, they use what's on hand (or foot).[1]

After the workshop, EtShalom began spreading the word about the hazards of conventional FemCare and promoting the use of alternatives. As a junior counselor at a summer camp, she led a cloth menstrual pad–making workshop. This was a turning point, EtShalom recalls: "The workshop was so popular that I led it every Saturday afternoon for two summers. My campers got really excited about it and starting asking me lots of questions about periods and vaginas, and I couldn't answer all of them so I started looking up answers. Thus began my career as a menstrual activist."[2]

At twenty-six, EtShalom is originator and owner of a small cloth menstrual pad business (the pads are called Rad Rags) and an online resource center for information on sexual, genital, and reproductive health, Below the Belt. She also writes a zine, *Owner's Manual: The Personal, the Political*, whose second issue includes articles titled "Adventures with Genital Warts," "The Death of a Yeast Infection," "Cramp Relief," and "How to Make Pads." For several years, EtShalom worked as a genital model for medical students in a Philadelphia hospital, giving trainees a hands-on experience performing gynecological exams under her direction, teaching them to examine their future patients with sensitivity and accuracy.

EtShalom is among those who populate the radical menstruation wing of the menstrual activism movement. I first encountered this enterprising activist during her workshop tour of college campuses, community centers, and living rooms in thirty-six cities between January and May 2004. Traveling exclusively via Greyhound, EtShalom did workshops on menstrual health, self-defense, and genital self-exam, enlightening more than four hundred people about the pleasures and possibilities of DIY menstrual care.

I was one of those four hundred. I met EtShalom at the Boston Skillshare, a punk-inspired DIY event held annually on the campus of Simmons College in Boston. I attended one of the many skill-building sessions on offer, a "Make Your Own Menstrual Pads" workshop, whose organizer sheepishly admitted from the outset that she "really didn't know much about why tampons and pads were bad for you."[3] EtShalom, also in attendance, graciously offered that she "knew a little bit" and launched into a well-informed litany of reasons to avoid commercial products (remarkably, without hijacking the event). I took in the scene, a small group of punk youth seated on the floor of a carpeted classroom, on my left a basket of cloth scraps, crude patterns, and needles and thread. As EtShalom engaged us in a discussion of why cloth pads like the ones we began to sew were preferable to conventional products, I realized that this is what a DIY workshop is all about: a few supplies, someone with a little know-how, someone else with a little rationale, and a group of eager learners. For punks, the project is rooted in a firm belief: It is better if we turn our back on corporate America and do it ourselves. This has surely been EtShalom's inspiration as she has developed a reputation as expert and resource to many.

A few days later, I attended a menstrual health and politics workshop EtShalom conducted on my own campus at the University of Massachusetts

Boston Women's Center. The workshop was not dissimilar from the one at the Skillshare, except this time EtShalom was officially at the helm and attendees—a wider mix of folks, some punk identified and some not—were a bit more passive. Undaunted, EtShalom confidently laid out the health, environmental, and social implications of conventional FemCare, emphasizing the ways the FemCare industry exploits consumers and endangers their health and the environment. Then she passed a stack of precut cloth, patterns, and needles and thread and introduced menstrual care alternatives as we began making our own reusable pads.

What is most memorable to me about that workshop is the flap just before the event. The event organizer, aware of my connection to EtShalom, contacted me to ask, "Is EtShalom a woman or not?" EtShalom, then at the beginning of her transition from woman to genderqueer, had requested that the marketing materials for the workshop not use female pronouns when referring to "her." For the organizer, the ambiguity was troubling and its implications complicated. Was it appropriate to have someone who did not identify as a woman lead a workshop on menstruation? (The assumption that a person identifying as a woman is necessarily an appropriate presenter for such a topic—and that someone who does not so identify is not—is also problematic).

EtShalom was born Shira, briefly changed her name to Shix as she began transitioning from a gender identity of girl/woman to her present expression as genderqueer and ultimately claimed the name Yonah. This complicates more than just pronoun use. (I use from this point on "squee" and "squir," terms EtShalom invented to replace "s/he" and "her/his," when referring to EtShalom.) Even before EtShalom's transition, squee has long been invested in providing health-care information sensitive to the needs of diverse people, presenting material in a transinclusive way. Punk identified and informed by a third-wave feminist sensibility, EtShalom takes squir toolkit on the road, critiquing the corporate FemCare establishment while teaching others to do it themselves. I urged the event organizer to edit the advertising copy according to EtShalom's wishes and allow the workshop planning to proceed. The event was a success.

THE IDEOLOGICAL INSPIRATIONS
OF RADICAL MENSTRUATION

That EtShalom, a biological woman turned genderqueer, is doing menstrual activism is significant, for it is one key to the uniqueness of the second (and larger) of the two dominant wings of the contemporary menstrual activism movement, the radical menstruation wing (forty-three of the sixty-five activists I interviewed fell into this category). While there are similarities between the two wings, the differences between them are most striking. Radical menstruationists challenge not only the menstrual status quo, skewering in particular the commercial industry they blame for disease and pollution, but also the dichotomous gender structure at the root of gender-based oppression. In contrast, feminist-spiritualists embrace menstruation as a meaningful experience unique to women and fore-ground their identity as women who menstruate. Radical menstruation activists uncouple the gendered body from menstruation. Women who menstruate become "menstruators." Assumptions about *who* menstruates are challenged. Inspired by third-wave values of multiplicity, contradiction, inclusion, and everyday feminism, these menstrual activists do DIY public health on a small scale at the same time they queer or disturb the gender divide.

Like the feminist-spiritualists, radical menstruation activists reject the characterization of menstruation as a shameful, useless hassle best kept hidden from view, even from menstruators themselves. Unlike the feminist-spiritualists, however, these activists largely reject a romanticized view of menstruation. While they resist the menstrual taboo, most stop short of elevating the bodily process to the status of spiritual experience. Their more pragmatic view is represented by one activist who said, "You don't have to mythologize for it to be okay. It is all right in its own right. It is blood. Period. We bleed." In this view, menstruation is neither a gift nor a curse; it is a bodily process understood as the object of corporate colonization, and it is time to take it back.

Environmentalism

What drew these activists to the issue of menstruation in the first place? What movements led them to a critical evaluation of dominant menstrual attitudes and practices? Several of the activists made explicit the joint influence of feminism and environmentalism as progenitors of menstrual activism. Arguing for the wide reach of menstrual activism, campus activist and organizer of an Anti-Tampon Conference in 2000, Kristin Garvin: "I think that for an issue to really motivate you to act it has to hit you on some really personal level and you can't get much more personal than this. It's such crucial subject matter because it has such potential to empower womyn and change their lives. I felt it was also a great campaign because it addressed very important feminist and environmental issues at the same time and not many campaigns brought these two movements or interests together so obviously."[4]

Similarly, Courtney Dailey, one of the Bloodsisters' founders, reported that "environmentalism and feminism brought me to this issue." For her, the connections run even deeper; she links radical menstruation with wider struggles for "human rights," against capitalism, racism, classism, homophobia, heterosexism, sizeism, ableism, the list goes on: "I think that all these struggles ask us to pay closer attention to our lives, and the way we live, understanding that how we live directly affects other people in our communities and in our world. Assessing our privilege, understanding where it comes from, and trying to make changes in our lives that may have effects that reach beyond what we can imagine, these are all part of our common struggles, I hope."[5] adee, another founder of Bloodsisters and its principal activist, elaborated on the intersecting inspirations for the group in an e-mail to me on June 9, 2009:

> We need the entire spectrum of spectrums to create change and value and respect every manifestation—"the second wave," the anarchists of 1960s campus rising, the environments, the radical feminist art history in the 70s, the black panthers, the riot grrls addressing sexism and racism in male-dominated punk/music scene, the Zapatistas, the african women not switching to tampons, economics of socially conscious small business, the genderization of authority/respect, seattle demo/ quebec city demo, colonialist constructs of cleanliness and "woman" and "primitive," [and] the very obvious shift in advertisement showing "new blood" in the executive suites that have made the recent change in making such campaigns more trendy/modern/speaking a language for teenagers.

The inspirations adee lists, however, are markedly more robust than most I heard during my fieldwork. Most of the activists' stories of initial attraction to menstrual issues were similar to Dailey's. Initially drawn to the environmental movement, they grew disillusioned with what they saw as environmentalism's inattentiveness to structural sources of oppression. Dailey first learned about the dioxin-tampon link in high school in the early 1990s through environmentalism. Once educated, she was compelled to act: "I was alarmed and knew that I had to do something, to tell people about this serious problem and how they could avoid one more carcinogenic thing in their lives." But over time, she grew dissatisfied with the shortsightedness of the environmentalists in her community: "The environmental folks I was hanging around had an analysis of the world in these green terms that were leaving out essential parts of systems and structures that I was beginning to understand as oppressive. I was beginning to think that there needed to be more radical, not reformist, ideas about society."[6]

Dailey found what she was looking for in feminism, an ideology and a practice that wove together analyses of class, race, gender, and sexuality in ways that made sense to her. But the feminism she found was a different breed than that of a previous generation, and it departed sharply from the feminism that informs the feminist-spiritualists' wing of the menstrual activism movement.

Third-Wave Feminism and Antiessentialism

Third-wave feminism produces a particular feminist identity that in turn shapes a menstrual politics marked as much by what it is not as by what it is. According to Carol Church, the writer of the now defunct e-zine *Whirling Cervix*, as menstrual activists, third-wave feminists are not "the type to enthuse about becoming one with the chalice and the Goddess."[7] Her words reveal an intentional dissociation from the cultural feminist celebration of the body, the goddess, and all things natural and earthy so fundamental to feminist-spiritualist menstrual activism. In some cases, this disenchantment with goddess-inspired menstrual politics manifested as outright hostility. For instance, journalist Karen Houppert narrates her encounter with alternative menstrual products in her 1995 *Village Voice* feature article "Embarrassed to Death: The Hidden Dangers of the Tampon Industry":

> My foray into the world of alternative menstrual products takes the shape of a super hero's quest. Special powers: a death-defying ability to contort my vagina around recalcitrant products. Shazam! An unruly sponge is tamed. Holy nappies! One more double-thick pad is wrestled into submission beneath jeans. My mission: to make the world safe for femi-nazis. My motto: no super plus is too great, no junior/lite too insignificant. Only one thing can bring me to my knees. The Kryponite of the body-and-blood set: celebrate-our-cycles liturgy. Sadly, New Ageans dominate this market. Take New Cycle Products for example. The catalogue cover looks innocuous enough. Just another sea nymph dangling from a slivered moon. But inside affirmations—"May our sunlight-consciousness illuminate the vessel of our moon-womb-chalice"—attack me from all directions. Moon Bowls, pots to soak used pads in before washing them and returning this "rich soaking water" to plants and gardens for "amazing results," reinforce the over-riding theme: "Women have an innate understanding of the Universe that is directly linked to their ability to cycle." And catalogue copy is not content with your cycles. It wants your first-born as well. First timers are sucked into celebrating menarche with the "Cycle Celebration Crown Kits."[8]

As this narrative suggests, radical menstruation activists, who overwhelmingly identify with third-wave feminism (not always by name, but often through discourse and actions), do not necessarily identify with a woman-as-nurturer representation. Embedded in a historical postmodern moment of cultural relativism, categorizations of any sort are suspect, especially given how race, class, sexuality, and other layers of identity make any monolithic conception of woman (or anyone) impossible. Rather, third-wave feminists argue that contradiction is the stuff of women's experience that must be incorporated into any feminist analysis and practice. In the introduction to her edited anthology *To Be Real: Telling the Truth and Changing the Face of Feminism*, Rebecca Walker points out: "Constantly measuring up to some cohesive fully down-for-the-feminist-cause identity without contradictions and messiness and lusts for power and luxury items is not a fun or easy task. . . . For many of us it seems that to be a feminist in the way that we have seen or understood feminism is to conform to an identity and way of living that doesn't allow for individuality or complexity or less than perfect personal histories."[9]

Gender-based separatism as a means to build women's community and provide safe spaces for women to explore, question, and heal from the ravages of sexism is anathema to third-wave feminists. Third-wavers generally remain unconvinced that so-called women's culture has caused significant change in the gender order. Besides, third-wave feminists argue, we need to build more alliances with progressive men and make room for gender-variant people, not sever already too-weak ties and perpetuate exclusionary rigid definitions of identity. In particular, one can't expect women of color or poor women to deny their race or class and identify only as women—a reduction that ignores the ways that racism and classism, for example, shape identity and experience. For socially marginalized women, connections to men of color or to poor men can be essential for survival and solidarity.

Finally, cultural feminist–inspired spiritualist discourse often links menstruation with reproduction, an equation that does not add up for women who do not identify with their procreative capacities (or lack of capacities). Calling attention to the uniquely female experience of monthly bleeding also excludes young girls; postmenopausal, transgendered, transsexual, and intersex women; and women who for myriad other reasons cannot bleed—a point EtShalom hastens to make through speaking and writing. Third-wave feminists are invested in inclusion, multiplicity, and contradiction, not essentialism, and thus find cultural feminism ideologically rigid and backward.

This conceptual divide may explain why the movement has sprouted two wings. The differences are profound, and there is little cross-fertilization going on between the parts of the whole. However, a few activists represent a hybrid of the disparate approaches to menstrual activism, for example, self-described tattoo artist, zinester, and witch Hag Rag, who operates a web-based menstrual pad business and sells both goddess soap (in the shape of Venus of Willendorf) and pads and blankets fashioned of fabric printed with skulls.[10] More commonly, however, radical menstruation activists explicitly distance themselves from what they perceive as soft, sappy, or mystical yet admit that menstrual cycle awareness offers real benefits. For example, Marie Abbondanza, author of the zine *It's Your Fucking Body #2*: Reclaim Your Cunt, confessed: "For me, personally, making my own pads and using the keeper has created so much more intimacy between me and my menstruating cunt. That sounds really granola-womyn-dykey but it's true for me at least." In the same publication, regarding the making and washing of reusable cloth pads, Abbondanza struggles with representation and reality: "I don't really know what I'm trying to say here and I'm desperately attempting to not sound really cheesy and wombmoon-ly, but I think there is a definite value to radical menstruation because it breaks down those sterile walls of individually wrapped plastic devices that keep us from becoming friends with our vaginas."[11]

"It all comes from that place that punk's been"

When I asked Bloodsister Emily Biting to comment on the origins of radical menstruation, she said: "It all comes from that place that punk's been. It's a third-wave, kick-butt aesthetic. DIY's a big part. Definitely anarchist leanings. Anarcha feminist politics. As in trying to be nonhierarchical. It is hard to sort out, but it all has the same mom."[12] While Biting admits that the roots of radical menstruation are tangled, her musings on its influences were reiterated by many others I interviewed. Repeatedly in my study, DIY, a key component of the punk lifestyle, surfaced as central to radical menstruation. In fact, DIY is the backbone of radical menstruation.

The punk movement dates to the alternative music scene in the late 1960s in North America and the 1970s in the United Kingdom. Much more than music, punk is a lifestyle informed by a particular social analysis. According to an ethnographer of girls' punk subculture, Lauraine Leblanc: "There is little agreement about [punk's] geographic origins, its ideologies, its membership, and even . . . its continued existence."[13] There is agreement, however, that punk began as a subculture based on music that more generally enacted a disgruntled and direct opposition to authority and mainstream culture. Rather than subscribing to the norms of compliance and obedience expected of youth, punks—including those who subscribe to types labeled hardcore, Spirit of '77, gutter, crusty, postcard, new school, and old school—embrace stylized norms of opposition as members of a reflexive subculture, seeking "to remain outside the dominant culture, while illuminating central features of it."[14] Further, it is agreed that punk all along has existed as an overwhelmingly white subculture, which may explain the overwhelming whiteness of the radical menstruation wing.

DIY first materialized as a form of self-reliance when punks picked up guitars and taught each other how to play. According to Craig O'Hara, author of an insider's look into punk culture, *Philosophy of Punk: More than Noise!* the DIY ethic in the punk music scene originated as a means to resist the commercial music world, which was widely denigrated by punks for putting profits above all else. Selling out by musicians was anathema to punks, making DIY the only viable alternative. Thus punks created their own garage bands, both in defiance of corporatized music and as a matter of survival, since commercial record labels did not pick up punk music, at least in the United States.[15]

But punk DIY became more than that. It embodies a relentless scrutiny of mainstream culture and becomes a means to resist any number of its dominant values and practices. As one punk put it, "Punk taught me to question everything."[16] In the early days of the subculture, punk was synonymous with nihilism and indiscriminate consumption of drugs and alcohol. But as it aged, its "question everything" sensibility has meant rebelling against drugs, alcohol, and unfettered consumption; many punks have adopted veganism, a diet that includes no animal or animal-derived products.[17] Ted Leo, a punk musician, linked punk and veganism with "being poison free."[18] Becoming vegan, or its less extreme cousin, vegetarian, became a way to protest factory farms and animal cruelty—an affront to the speciesism foundational to contemporary attitudes about what is consumable and why.

The convergence of environmentalism, third-wave feminism, and punk produces the ideological inspiration that propels the radical menstruation movement, a frame that construes menstruation as a bodily process shaped by consumerism and controlled by corporations that disregard both human and environmental health. Consequently, the radical menstruation activists, skeptical, self-sufficient, and critical of mainstream culture, advocate that each menstruator take control back from corporations.

"Taking Control of Our Blood"

The Bloodsisters are widely considered the leaders of the radical menstruation movement. Founded in 1995 by adee, Courtney Dailey, and others, the Bloodsisters joined aesthetic sensibility with pointed political analysis to produce actions and materials that challenged the menstrual status quo, as their website suggests:

> Bloodsisters is an exciting launching pad girl base fueling action to combat the silence surrounding our female bodies
> we are girls using our own feminine protection to work against the corporate and cultural constructions of menstruation
> we are concerned with the serious health, environmental and psychological ramifications of the toxic feminine hygiene industry and are fighting to stop the whitewash on all fronts
> born out of a guerrilla girl recyclable pad distribution network, we are an ever growing group generating more creative projects to raise awareness surrounding menstrual girl-body politics
> these include publishing zines, weaving a web girl network, terrorizing bathroom walls, giving healthy health workshops, organizing art exhibits, distributing affordable, alternative products, sharing n boycotting, tabling n lobbying, stitching n bitching and always with winged power.[19]

Appropriating the language of the FemCare industry, the Bloodsisters reclaim the notions of protection and wings (a reference to menstrual pads fitted with adhesive wings) and assert that menstruators are in control of menstruation, not corporate interests that exploit and reinforce a cultural construction of menstruation as a curse to be managed.

Brackin "Firecracker" Camp, activist and cocreator of the zine *Femmenstruation Rites Rag* (with Chantel Guidry), told me that menstrual issues are a tangible application of the feminist theory she read in college in two women's studies courses. The potential influence of college training, especially in women's and gender studies, is great among those affiliated with the radical menstruation wing of the movement. All the activists in this population I interviewed attended college, and 69 percent of them took at least one women's or gender studies course during that time. Camp illustrated the meaningful connection between her education and her activism: "I could see myself in all the articles we were reading and analyze my reactions and opinions on both theoretical and actual levels." This education, made real through menstrual awareness, operates as a sort of gateway to a more comprehensive control of one's life. According to Camp: "Once we take control of issues around our blood, then we can be much more accepting and aware of our own bodies in other ways such as when a person makes a choice to have a baby then they are much more likely to make decisions regarding the birth that are better for them and the baby."[20]

The theme of taking control is perhaps the most pervasive in the discourse of radical menstruation. Without control, the activists explained, people are vulnerable to inhabiting a body alienated from the self, a body co-opted by corporate interests, a body disciplined by consumer culture. And when menstruators assert control over their own menstrual experience, they may feel enabled to live more whole lives. As Dailey enthused: "Helping women to know that they can take control of their menstruation back from scientists and multinational corporations is very exciting, as it can lead to thinking about taking back a lot of power, as well as planting seeds of critical thinking about the world and how we live in it."[21]

"Taking control" is expressed not only in the abstract. The radical menstruation activists are very clear that menstruators must disentangle themselves from the FemCare industry, first, by casting a critical eye on industry practices and products and, second, by teaching others how to, as one activist put it, "break the tampon addiction" through boycotts of conventional products, especially those produced by multinational corporations. Their objective is not to reform the industry (which is the aim of most boycotts) but to turn their back on it, for good. Paradoxically, they engage corporate structures through disengagement.

If the state has abrogated its role as a protector of public health and safety through federal agencies like the FDA and CDC, it figures minimally in menstrual activist discourse; not one activist I interviewed mentioned the state as implicated in producing, reinforcing, or benefiting from the dominant social construction of menstruation. Even when legislative action is proposed, radical menstruation activists seems less than enthused. The Robin Danielson Act (H.R. 5181), named after a woman who died of TSS, has failed to make any progress in Congress since its introduction in 1997. The bill, introduced by New York Representative Carolyn Mahoney, directs the National Institutes of Health (NIH) to conduct research to assess the safety of tampons (and asks the CDC to collect and report TSS information). The bill has been reintroduced four times since 1997, most recently in the 110th congressional session in 2008.[22] The few times I heard this bill mentioned during my fieldwork, the information was scant and suggestions regarding how to support the bill's progress through Congress never stipulated. Could the bill's poor track record be in part the result of activist inattention?

The activists set their sights not on the government but on the FemCare industry. What is it about the makers of single-use tampons and pads (and related products, such as "feminine wipes") that raises the ire of those affiliated with the radical menstruation wing?

A BRIEF PROFILE OF THE FEMCARE INDUSTRY

In 2005 the global FemCare industry amassed $17 billion in sales for tampons (15.1 percent), pads (69.4 percent), panty liners (15.2 percent), and feminine hygiene wipes (0.3 percent).[23] According to the 2006 "Feminine Hygiene Products—Global Strategic Business Report," which provides separate comprehensive analytics for the industry throughout the world and profiles 134 companies, the FemCare industry is expanding globally, mainly due to growth in "emerging markets."[24] In 2005 the U.S. FemCare industry reported approximately $2.3 billion in sales, but projections indicate a slight decline over the coming years, with a sales volume of $2.2 billion forecast for 2010. The anticipated decline in the U.S. market is mainly attributed "to significant demographic changes in the years ahead, when more women of the baby boom generation pass through menopause."[25]

In the United States, four players dominate the FemCare market: Procter & Gamble (P&G), makers of Tampax and Always; Kimberly-Clark (K-C), makers of Kotex and Poise (the latter is a product for incontinence); Johnson & Johnson (J&J), makers of OB and Stayfree; and Playtex Products, makers of Playtex.[26] All four companies produce and market a variety of consumer or medical goods in addition to their menstrual care products. P&G, K-C, and J&J have extensive multinational operations, and even Playtex sees markets outside North America as central to its growth strategy.

The Big Four—or "the corporate creeps," as some refer to these industry leaders—maintain or increase profits in the stagnant U.S. market by vying for market share through advertising, trying to convince consumers to use "innovative" products that have a higher profit margin, and capitalizing on trends in consumer attitudes, among other strategies. In their quest for market share companies of course advertise the quality and performance aspects of their products, such as the proper level of absorbency to meet needs or increase ease of use. But they also appeal to and reinforce the menstrual taboo, activists contend. For instance, Tampax's homepage carries the tag line "Tampax—Made to Go

Unnoticed," and Kotex came up with its "specially-designed rustle-free wrapper because there's no need to shout about it."[27]

Product innovation is admittedly ambiguous. At times the emphasis is more on repackaging than on offering new product functionality. According to a senior "private label" (in-store brand) executive, repackaging presents an opportunity for "taking a price increase by reducing the tampon count in . . . packages." Another executive explained why repackaging is essential: "P&G is leading a trend with Tampax Pearl—the category focus is moving from functional products to more cosmetic-appealing products. Tampax Pearl comes in a smaller, thinner, glossier tube with upgraded wrappers and packaging. When you're trading up a consumer by thirty percent on price, you have to dress it up."[28]

That a shift to "more cosmetic-appealing products" (including those that include plastic applicators, like Tampax's successful Pearl) may have an environmentally negative impact does not appear to be a concern of industry marketing professionals. As a matter of fact, all players seem eager to jump on the plastics bandwagon: "We're seeing dramatic growth in plastic. . . . Private label is in the game and capitalizing on it," enthuses a senior company representative in a trade publication.[29] In another trade mouthpiece, an industry observer makes it unmistakably clear that environmental sustainability is not among market priorities: "Unless you live in a more ecologically aware area, most people want a feminine hygiene product that has a good reputation for quality and a reasonable price. . . . If the product is also biodegradable and good for the environment, that will definitely help, but having a high quality level and a good price will be more important than environmental-friendliness in the long run."[30]

The FemCare industry's reputation for neglecting women's health (recall P&G's Rely tampon tragedy of the early 1980s) is further evidenced in this striking statement found in a trade publication: "Tampons are expected to decline the least . . . as an increasing number of consumers choose tampons above sanitary pads. Younger consumers who are becoming more dominant in the market are more knowledgeable about tampons and less fearful of Toxic Shock Syndrome (TSS) . . . . Expect manufacturers to push for teenage consumers through television and print advertisements, promotional partnerships with companies popular with teenagers and packaging intended to draw a female teenager's eye."[31]

Activists interpret such approaches as exploitative, taking advantage of girls' relative fearlessness, which may be attributable as much to ignorance as to the reality of product safety. Today's girls did not grow up with the tampon-related TSS outbreak of 1980, after all. But although products have changed somewhat, TSS remains a concern (and products are still mandated to carry TSS warning labels). Industry-attributed phrases such as "less fearful of TSS" feed the suspicions of the menstrual activists that the industry is downplaying (if not completely ignoring) the health hazards associated with tampon use. Given a disregard for the negative environmental implications of single-use products and an expressed strategy of charging more money for the same product in a snazzier box, all while the multinationals are spreading into "emerging markets," the FemCare industry is easy to hate from the activists' vantage point. They channel this hatred into resistance by turning their backs and doing without. For them, it is futile to attempt to work with industry representatives or government officials whose job it is to regulate FemCare. This sense of futility, I found, is rooted in pervasive distrust. The logic of radical menstruation activists is simple: Why try to talk to them when they can't even be trusted?

TURNING OUR BACKS ON THE BIG FOUR

Reform is pointless.

During my fieldwork, I repeatedly heard this sentiment expressed in a variety of ways. For example, I observed a discussion (more accurately, a rant) about the FemCare industry among a small group of young college students, who collectively listed the injustices and offenses committed by makers of conventional FemCare products: shaming women through ad campaigns, polluting air and water supplies, and producing products that cause microlacerations of the vaginal walls. To my surprise, someone added: "And there's that ridiculous packaging— what's up with this stupid labeling they've got on their boxes? Typical corporate behavior. What a racket. Who cares how many grams a tampon can absorb? Who even knows what a gram is? That's really stupid." This young activist, in spite of her passion for menstrual health and politics, operates unaware of the activism that precedes her. The stupid labeling to which she refers is the outcome of ten years of negotiations and consumer mobilization campaigns. Even if she knew the history of her movement, I predict that she would not revise her assessment. For the radical menstruation activists, reformist measures are inadequate, even wrongheaded. If you can't trust the corporations, you certainly cannot negotiate with them. There is no point in engaging with the Big Four. For the activists, true radical change requires not treating the symptoms but going to the root cause of corporate self-interest: capitalism itself.

A second story further illustrates this point. During my fieldwork, in early 2005, I sat in on a meeting during the Student Environmental Action Coalition's (SEAC) annual National Convergence—a series of meetings that gather representatives from SEAC member schools nationwide to educate them about the organization's campaigns. I joined the group of students interested in the Tampaction campaign, an initiative designed to educate students about the environmental, social, and health consequences of conventional FemCare and to encourage them to press campus bookstores to carry alternative products.[32]

During the session, a number of the students raised questions about conventional tampon safety. Some expressed confusion about the dioxin risk since the industry has changed its bleaching methods.[33] Others asked if there was solid evidence linking yeast infections, endometriosis, and microlacerations of the vaginal walls to tampon use. "What about TSS?" one asked. "How common is it today?" The leaders admirably fielded these questions, admitting that reliable data are not available, since most studies of FemCare products have been conducted by their manufacturers. There is a conflict of interest, they remarked.

When a student asked, "How do the companies answer these questions?" I spoke up: "If you want to hear it directly from them, I can put you in touch with representatives of the FemCare division at Procter & Gamble." All heads turned toward me. I explained that I had met with P&G reps during my research and when SEAC's campaign was mentioned during our conversation (perhaps not surprisingly to many, P&G was fully aware of it), they asked me to let the SEACers know that they were willing to meet with them to address their concerns about tampon safety. My offer and explanation met silence. I pressed: "I know you aren't big fans of them, but you'd have the chance to confront them about what you don't like about their products and their marketing." After more silence, one of the campaign leaders spoke up: "I don't think so. What would be the point of that? I don't trust them anyway."

Again, as this story shows, the point of activism in the radical menstruation view is not taking corporations to task directly, but slowly undermining them through the use of alternative femcare. This activism seeks neither to accommodate nor to improve the products of those who profit from what the activists see as the denigration of women's bodies. The point is, as the Bloodsisters artfully phrased it, to stop "riding the ol' cotton pony."

THE REVOLUTIONARY POTENTIAL
OF RADICAL MENSTRUATION

A radical view of menstruation is the foundation of the activism of both wings of the movement. That is, both incorporate a critique of the dominant cultural narrative of menstruation and promote alternative framings united by a refusal to exploit women's bodies. The radical menstruation activists' plan to take corporations down departs notably from the feminist-spiritualists, who center their efforts on the transformation of menstrual consciousness (though many do choose to use alternative menstrual products).

But from that point, the wings diverge. The feminist-spiritualists frame menstruation as a spiritually endowed, women-centered experience that unites all women. The radical menstruation activists judge the feminist-spiritualist project of self-transformation limited because it fails to touch the corporate structures that disempower menstruators. L. A. Kauffman, writer and radical activist, asserts that movements that tend toward individual-level self-transformation frame human struggles as the product of a change in attitude, for which the remedy is a further attitude change. Approaching social inequality this way, according to Kauffman, diverts attention from addressing how systems of power and privilege produce disadvantage. Biting, a member of the Bloodsisters collective, commented on the feminist-spiritualist approach to menstrual activism: "Painting yourself with blood and dancing under the moon isn't activism. It's narcissistic. Well, let me revise that: It's individualistic."[34]

Here Biting implies a distinction between individualistic (or self-centered) actions and individual actions as a means to effect social change. Indeed, her critique of the feminist-spiritualists echoes my own in the previous chapter: The feminist-spiritualists engage a partial form of life politics at the everyday level but fail, ultimately, to translate personal struggles into bids for social transformation. The radical menstruation activists, in contrast, succeed at life politics as conceived by social theorist Anthony Giddens. They act personally but think globally, attempting through individual change to radically alter the consumption practices that sustain advanced capitalism.

Imagine the contrast between women sharing their moontime in a makeshift Red Tent and a group of punk college students sewing their own cloth menstrual pads on the floor of their residence hall common area. Both events presume that social change starts with the individual. Both manifest a commitment to an alternative view of the menstruating body and refuse to banish menstruation to a private world of shame and secrecy. In these ways, both approaches are radical, going to the source of profoundly negative attitudes regarding a normal bodily process. But for the feminist-spiritualists, the change begins and ends with the individual, though the intention may be grander. Because the feminist-spiritualists frame menstruation using a cultural feminist analysis of womanhood, the tactics that emerge are limited in their appeal and ultimately reduce social change to personal transformation.

The radical menstruation activists draw from punk, third-wave feminism, and environmentalism to resist corporate control of the body. Their strategy of making menstrual pads and alerting others to the hazards of conventional FemCare is designed, as a longtime activist told me, "to cut off the head of the capitalist beast and kick it in the groin."[35] The intent is to mobilize consumer power in a boycott of toxic polluting products. Because their activism combines critique with a plan of structural change enacted in the everyday, it is both radical and revolutionary.

Radical menstruation also diverges from the social change agenda of the previous generation of menstrual activists—the feminist health activists, environmentalists, and consumer rights advocates who united in the 1980s to hold the FemCare industry accountable for women's health and safety. Menstrual activists at that time focused aggressively on reform, not on radical structural change. When activists pushed for uniform absorbency ratings of tampons, they were trying to improve the existing FemCare industry (and the government that regulates it) and in turn impact millions of women. But when they put on suits and flew to Washington, D.C., to confront industry and government representatives, their actions did not aggressively attack the idea of the "necessity" of tampons and the menstrual taboo that constructs the need for so-called disposable products designed to render menstruation invisible. In fact, by working tirelessly to improve the safety profile of single-use products, they reified menstruation as a process best cleaned up and tidied away, even if more safely.

Nevertheless, after ten years of protracted struggle, in 1992 the activists won: Standardized tampon absorbency ratings were adopted industrywide. But when the next generation of activists came of age, they did not continue this struggle but engaged in wholesale rejection of entities they continue to view as beyond reform. Radical menstruation activists, troubled by the rise of global capitalism and consumerism run amok, position the multinational corporation in the crosshairs. Yet they take aim through a strategy of disengagement.

TACTICS: SEEING THE SECOND WAVE IN THE THIRD

In *Different Wavelengths: Studies of the Contemporary Women's Movement*, editor Jo Reger suggests that "the challenge for contemporary feminism is to take a look at past waves (or at least campaigns, organizations, protests, and sit-ins) and uncover the relationship between past and present. Feminist history provides insight into the roots of current ideology and strategy." Reger also points out that a change in feminist ideology today "corresponds to a change in tactics with third-wave activism characterized as computer generated, do it yourself (DIY), online and in cyberspace."[36] I certainly agree that access to computer technology has transformed activism, but I do not view the tactics—at their heart—as fundamentally different from those we associate with the second-wave. The form may be different, but the content is familiar.

It is easy to be distracted by technological innovation, but if we peel away the novelty, we see personal narrative, disarming humor, and street theater present in both waves. As some second-wavers hasten to point out, similarities across the movements and historical continuity are lost on many contemporary young feminists. Lisa Maria Hogeland, for example, argues that generational formulations of feminist difference as divisive and destructive (and an evasion of the true political divide between consciousness and social change) are hardly innovative: "The in-your-face activist style of Riot Grrrls and other young(er) feminists is, however, neither unique nor specific to a younger generation of feminists; it bears, in fact, quite marked similarities to some early second-wave activities. But young(er) feminists too often don't know much about the zap-actions, the mimeographed flyer, and the materiality of early second-wave protest."[37] While I do not share Hogeland's unequivocal denial of an emergent feminism that offers something new, I see her point. Tactically speaking, at least, many of the tools and actions deployed by third-wave feminists are reinventions. Self-help may now manifest as DIY and mimeographed manifestos may now take the form of zines, but at their root the tactics of the previous wave have survived into the twenty-first century. I am especially committed to making clear these connections because I found historical ignorance among the radical menstruation activists I met. Like the activist who dismissed the tampon absorbency ratings as "stupid," nearly all were unaware of the work of women's health and consumer advocates who toiled in the late 1970s and throughout the 1980s. They seemed unaware of the history I mapped in chapter three (indeed, as I wrote that history, I often imagined them as my audience). I was struck by their assumption that menstrual activism is a third-wave creation particular to the punk scene, for instance, or an outgrowth of the contemporary environmental movement. While these influences shape menstrual activism, its history goes much deeper and reaches much further into the history of feminist organizing of the 1970s. Tactically speaking, menstrual activism draws from a rich and varied legacy of feminist agitation.

Zines: The Power of a Sharpie and a Photocopier

According to zine historian Stephen Duncombe, these modest but mighty periodicals were born in the 1930s when fans of science fiction began producing "fanzines" to communicate with each other as consumers, critics, and producers of science fiction.[38] In the 1970s, fans of punk rock music started producing zines in which they discussed the genre and culture unique to punk. In the 1980s, when zine making was taken up by fans of myriad other cultural genres, alienated self-publishers ignored by the mainstream, and political dissenters from the 1960s and 1970s, the current generation of zines was born (and the "fan" was dropped).

Zines represent a punk value, corporate resistance in action. V. Vale, editor of *Zines!* asks:

> Why zines? They are a grassroots reaction to a crisis in the media landscape. What was formerly *communication* has become a fully implemented *control process*. Corporate-produced advertising, television programming and PR campaigns dictate the twenty-first century, "anything goes" consumer lifestyle. TV networks, newspapers and magazines have been taken over by a handful of business culture financiers who co-opt and exploit any emerging "youth revolt" as soon as it begins to manifest. The oft-lamented homogenizing effect of worldwide media is now a *reality*.[39]

In the hands of menstrual activists zines become health zines, intended for women (and others) who question corporately derived health data and seek other forms of information. In an analysis of fifty-eight woman-created zines and interviews with forty women zinesters conducted by Dawn Bates and Maureen McHugh, zines appeal to young women and serve as "a method of feminist empowerment and resistance." The self-created and controlled forum was particularly appealing to young women, the researchers report, because it enabled them to "exercise their voice." Zines are an alternative to mainstream fare such as teen magazines, which, M. J. Finders argues, acculturate girls into dominant economic ideology, whereas zines resist, both in form and content. Making the case that zines are the new feminist communication frontier, Ann Cvetkovich, herself a feminist scholar and zine maker, sees zines as "the house organ of a new generation of feminists. . . . Using the photocopy machine and the power of self-distribution, the zine maker does not need a publisher to get her word out. Feminist intellectuals waiting for the media to come calling might take a lesson here."[40]

Independent of rules of design, censors, or quality standards, zinesters can express themselves unfettered. Duncombe argues that zine writers, "alienated from mainstream political institutions, and wary of any constraint on their individuality" (a cornerstone of punk identity and action), "reject a strategic model of politics and communication entirely in the search for a more 'authentic' formula." The model of politics they embrace is a discourse of the individual. Expanding what counts as political, they personalize politics by filtering issues through daily lived experience. Often the "information is presented in a way that keeps it from being just another floating statistic in a sea of information."[41]

Nearly all zines are considered authentic media. Interestingly, while high-tech means are available to most contemporary zinesters, it is typical for zines to be handwritten and crudely assembled. The point is to eschew the glitz and gloss of corporate mass-produced material, generating instead a homespun and intimate look that sets the zine apart.

According to Duncombe and others, the culture of zines has grown dramatically.[42] Due to the ephemeral nature of any self-published and self-distributed product, however, it is difficult to pin down the number of zines in circulation, let alone track a growth curve. One zine researcher cited between ten and fifty thousand zines traded or sold to an estimated readership of one to three million.[43]

Nearly all radical menstrual activists in this study relied on zines for their information. Eight of the activists I interviewed created their own zines, another contributed to a zine, and the Bloodsisters created a series of zines, the widely circulated *Red Alert*. Through the course of my research, I collected thirty-five menstrual activist zines, each devoted exclusively to exposing hazards associated with conventional menstrual care and discussing alternatives. (There are numerous other zines on women's health, the punk scene, feminism, and anarchism that include a piece or two on the issue of menstrual activism, but my focus was on zines on the topic of menstruation.)

In my analysis, I found these materials followed a similar format, confirming Duncombe's observation of zines as a forum for "personalized politics." In most cases, the zines begin with an explanation of what's wrong with the conventional or mainstream FemCare industry in terms of hazards to women's health and devastation to the environment. Typically a detailed discussion of alternatives to mainstream commercial sanitary pads and tampons follows, often a narrative in which the writer shares her experiences with each alternative. Finally the zines typically provide a list of resources for further information—other zines, websites, and sources for purchasing alternative products. Sometimes the zine includes a pattern for making one's own reusable cloth menstrual pads. (One zine in my collection is exclusively devoted to this project.)

But zines do more than disseminate information as they push against institutional structure and norms. They also work to pull activists together. According to Bates and McHugh's analysis of third-wave feminist zines, zinesters use the medium to build community, or "network," in the more common parlance of zinesters.[44] Writers connect with readers who inspire writers who become activists who become writers and so on, slowly building a web. Menstrual activist zines similarly reference each other, reprinting articles and images, quoting passages, and suggesting related zines as resources. Miki Walsh's ubiquitous "Friends Don't Let Friends Use Tampons" bumper sticker pops up in numerous zines, as does Fawn P.'s "Anatomy of a Tampon" (which details the health and environmental effects, the profits of the Big Four, and an exhaustive list of tampon ingredients), Kristin Garvin's cloth-pad pattern, and excerpts from Inga Muscio's *Cunt: A Declaration of Independence*. In addition, a plethora of images and text from the Bloodsisters' zines find their way into the pages of other zines. It is clear that the zinesters are reading and relying on each other's work. This free sharing of ideas is facilitated by the Punk ethic of propertylessness (sometimes referred to as "copyleft"). Punk culture does not tolerate notions of ownership. Space, resources, and information are freely shared for the good of the group, so it follows that intellectual property such as zine content is fair game. In a rare acknowledgment of copyright infringement, the Bloodsisters state in one of their zines: "All images respectfully stolen." This ethic is an echo of 1960s and 1970s radical countercultural values and tactics (for example, Abbie Hoffman's 1971 *Steal This Book*).

Like the feminist-spiritualists who create and sustain a network via books, the zinesters comprise a web of activists learning from one another, even if only through written words and graphics. In this spirit, zinesters are eager to share their zines with one another. A typical response after reading a zine, I've found, is to send a note of gratitude and one's own zine, thus further promoting the cross-fertilization of ideas and resources. More often, zinesters sell their zines to recoup the cost of production, or they arrange some kind of trade. (I've seen zines exchanged for stamps and vegan cookies, for example.) Zinesters set up tables at zine fairs such as the annual Beantown Zinetown in Boston, and at band performances, rallies, demonstrations, college campuses, and outdoor festivals. But more often the work of distributing zines is outsourced to a third party, a distribution service (a "distro"). Typically small-scale DIY operations run by individuals or small groups, the distros catalogue their collections and operate via mail order; some of the more sophisticated offer searchable online databases. The existence of the distros (and new ones appear at a rapid rate) suggests the value placed on getting zines into the hands of readers, a desire for wide circulation also in evidence at punk shows, political events, and festivals, where zines are hot items for sale or trade.

Yesterday's Zines. When I give presentations on my work on menstrual activism, audience members are often charmed by the zines in my collection. Their raw energy, sassy language, and free association of image and word strike many as fresh and bold. But this informal, grassroots communication medium is hardly unique to contemporary menstrual activism, in line with Reger's argument that "much of what appears to be new today in contemporary feminism has it roots in the past." More specifically, she reminds us (with the help of a key second-wave figure): "In a precursor to the feminist zine . . . , second-wave feminists wrote treatises, analyses, children's stories, and manifestos, mimeographed them, and sent them around the country." Reger quotes Susan Brownmiller, who recalls that writing was central to the creation of community and the spreading of ideas in the 1960s and 1970s. As a result, women's newspapers sprang up around the country, largely published without access to printing presses. She describes one such newspaper, *Plexus*, as "typed with ragged right margins on an IBM Selectric and pasted up with rubber cement."[45]

Many of these mimeographed and hand-distributed feminist manifestos and newspapers were themselves influenced by the New Left and student movement organizations in which early women's liberationists had been participants, for example, *Sojourner: A Women's Forum*, which began as a sixteen-page newspaper serving the Massachusetts Institute of Technology community and blossomed into one of the most successful and widely read feminist newspapers in the United States. (It finally suspended publication in 2002.)[46] Another example comes from the Redstockings, a short-lived but famous radical feminist group founded in the late 1960s.[47] This group wrote in 1969 and published in 1975 the "Redstockings Manifesto," which identifies all men as oppressors and calls for the development of "female class consciousness through sharing experience and publicly exposing the sexist foundation of all our institutions." In 1968 Valerie Solanis wrote and mimeographed a fiery polemic, the *S.C.U.M. Manifesto*, which she sold on the street. The next year, the *Manifesto* was published by Olympia Press.[48]

In the fall of 1968, Joreen, a.k.a Jo Freeman, proposed in *The Bitch Manifesto* an organization to be called BITCH and composed of "bitches" (followed by a list of the characteristics some or all bitches possess). "A woman should be proud to declare she is a Bitch, because Bitch is Beautiful," Joreen states. "It should be an act of affirmation by self and not negation by others."[49] The piece was first published in *Notes from the Second Year*, edited by Firestone and Koedt, and reprinted and distributed in pamphlet form, approximating the style and reach of a contemporary zine.

Still another precursor of the feminist zine is the first edition of the international bestseller and bible of women's health, *Our Bodies, Ourselves* (now in its eighth revised edition). The groundbreaking work, which quickly became an underground success, began as *Women & Their Bodies*, a 138-page booklet printed on newsprint with handwritten text on its cover.

Websites and E-Zines. Not all radical menstruation activists are Luddites. Some readily embrace technology and mount their own websites, in some cases as a platform to make activist materials widely available. Sometimes these websites take the form of e-zines—electronic versions of paper zines (a little cleaner and a lot more accessible, but still punk). Their discourse contrasts sharply with corporate communication (marketing) and maintains the radical ethos of self-reliance and corporate resistance.

Menstrual activists cultivate awareness, or what one zinester called "familiarization," in a number of clever ways, continuing the second-wave feminist consciousness-raising legacy of promoting personalized social change. S.P.O.T., a website created and maintained by menstrual activist Tracy Bannett, uses the self as subject of study, sharing the results for everyone's benefit. Bannett posted journalist Karen Houppert's humorous personal account of trying each of several alternative products, including cloth pads, the Keeper, the Diva Cup, the Moon Cup, the Sea Sponge, chlorine-free disposable pads, and non-chlorine-bleached 100 percent cotton tampons.[50] Miki Walsh's website, Randomgirl, offers a similar tour of alternative menstrual products in a narrative that reads nothing like a series of commercials, but rather like personal testimonies that expose the pros and cons of using each product from one woman's perspective, experiences readers might consider as they embark on their own experiments.

This self-as-example or self-as-study approach enjoys a rich tradition in the history of second-wave feminist self-help. For instance, when Lorraine Rothman first developed and practiced menstrual extraction in the 1970s, she insisted on trying the controversial procedure on herself before offering it to others. As she traveled around the country teaching women to perform the procedure, the implication was that "if it's good enough for me, it's good enough for you."[51] When today's radical menstruation activists share their experiences, the tone sometimes seems at cross-purposes with promoting alternative menstrual care. But again, the aim is not persuasion as much as it is exposure. For example, Houppert's less-than-rousing endorsement of cloth pads that appears on the S.P.O.T. website grounds the trial of the new and alternative in personal and uncensored experience. Her objective is not to convince the reader that cloth pads are best, but to share her own experience with this option, including the negative. Here, in what she dubs "notes from her menstrual odyssey," Houppert discusses the utility of the reusable cloth pad: "Major bummer for the city dweller who hasn't got her own washer and dryer and sometimes doesn't do laundry for weeks at a time. Plus, it's very much a drag when you discover, a week or two after the fact, that you've forgotten a used pad, now buried and fermenting at the bottom of your gym bag. True, cloth pads are comfier and less bulky than commercially sold paper ones, but it's a little like comparing a corset with a girdle."[52]

This strategy of sharing personal experience—the good, the bad, and the ugly—reassures the reader that s/he is getting at least one woman's true account, in contrast to the slick advertising campaigns most of us must decode and decipher when making a product choice. The activists work hard at speaking consumer to consumer, and steer clear of painting a solely positive picture. Personal experiences are not sanitized here; they are real and messy and sometimes contradictory. "You, the reader, are smart enough to make your choices," goes the discourse, "and we refuse to insult your intelligence (and buy into the corporate model) by leading you to purchase a product that may not be right for you." As S.P.O.T. suggests on its home page: "Explore the site, read articles written by others, look at alternatives, and then make up your own mind."

At times, personal experience as a tool of decision making crosses the boundary to self-effacement, for instance, Miki Walsh's pen name, Randomgirl, which seems to imply that she is neither an expert nor attached to an institution, but just one girl with something to say. When she identifies herself on her website as a distributor of the Keeper, she undermines herself as the best source for this product, perhaps communicating her ambivalence about participating in the world of commerce: "And if you don't feel comfortable getting a Keeper from me, but you still want one, PLEASE check out Eco Logicque, Inc, which is the major distributor of The Keeper. You should definitely go and buy from them, if you feel funny mailing your payment to a little *Randomgirl* . . . or if you want to use a credit card . . . then again, they probably deserve your business more than I do regardless, 'cuz * they* were doing this when *I* was still running around wearing o.b.☺" In the same vein, Random Girl titled her 1997 webpage Random Girl Rambles about the Keeper, although she did little actual rambling and much dispensing of detailed, clearly organized information. Similarly, the e-zine *Whirling Cervix* heads the first of eleven well-organized and comprehensive pages of information, "I babble about menstruation," again suggesting that the reader take this text as nothing more than one individual's (ostensibly disorganized) take on one topic.

Diminishing the self as authority has two functions. First, making clear that the writer is just one Randomgirl, for instance, empowers the reader to value her (or his) own experiences and opinions. Critical thinking and personal exploration are modeled and championed: If I did this (resisted, experimented and even wrote a zine or website about it), so can you. The point is not to suppress free expression but to stimulate more of it.

The second related purpose of the tone of "little ol' me" is to mark a noticeable distance from so-called, often self-described experts who disempower women by dictating what is right and wrong and invite no dialogue (often in a tone of paternal reassurance). In the context of menstrual activism, public enemy number one is, of course, the FemCare industry. According to the activists, the obvious agenda of the marketers of the FemCare industry is to position themselves as knowing best what women need and want when it comes to managing menstruation. Activists do not perceive consumer empowerment or environmental responsibility as core corporate concerns. The activists resist what they view as corporate priorities and perhaps overcompensate by packaging their own message as individualized and one of many voices unafraid of, even encouraging, challenge. Aware of the threat of cooptation, they work hard to keep their distance from those they so passionately resist.

Finally, websites can supply activists with tools to spread awareness. Naomi Klein, author of the bestselling exposé of corporate branding NO LOGO, defines a fairly new form of activism, "culture jamming," as "the practice of parodying advertisements and hijacking billboards in order to drastically alter their messages."[53] Culture jammers, according to Klein, reject the passive absorption of advertising and transform the intended one-way flow of communication from advertiser to uncritical consumer to a "talk back" in which the consumer reveals the story beneath the advertisement. In 2000, Walsh, the Randomgirl, teamed up with another activist, Julia Stewart, to produce a series of posters based on a P&G advertising campaign of the late 1990s.

Walsh and Stewart jammed P&G's "Tampax Was There" campaign, which linked key cultural events, such as marathons, Woodstock, and feminist icons like Rosie the Riveter with the ever-reliable Tampax. The implication at work in the P&G campaign was this: Tampax has been protecting women through the years, through wars, sporting events, and the 1960s revolution. It is a liberated woman's best friend. Walsh and Stewart's ads use P&G's campaign language to expose—through irony—the FemCare giant's questionable practices and to suggest that Tampax is responsible for pollution and disease: "It was there all right and you wish it weren't."

Like the work of other culture jammers who take an anticonsumerist stance, Walsh and Stewart's ads can be seen as a type of consumer boycott.[54] Boycotts are increasingly media oriented, "seeking to have an effect by damaging the target's reputation."[55] Disparaging and thus undermining the dominance of the FemCare industry is precisely the aim of radical menstruation culture jammers.

Activist Chella Quint combines culture jamming and ad parody through her campaign for Skids, a faux "masculine hygiene product for when you are feeling less

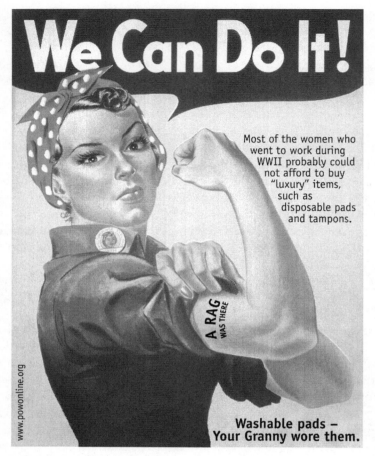

Figure 5. Miki Tapio Walsh and Julia D. Stewart, "Rosie the Riveter on the Rag," 2000. Courtesy of the artists.

than fresh!" The copy on the website, http://www.skidspads.co.uk/, is deceptively authentic:

> Skids is a sanitary product, just for guys! It's a way to keep our
>   private problems just between us.
> Totally discreet and disposable—to keep those nasty after-effects of drinking
>   too much beer to ourselves, and away from the ladies.
> Skids is a masculine hygiene product specially designed to follow a man's
>   contours and curves—perfect for when you're having one of *'those'*
>   nights.
> Now you can avoid the shame and embarrassment usually caused by the fear
>   of someone finding our your *'little secret.'*

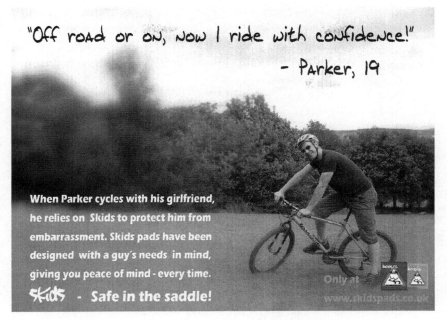

Figure 6. Chella Quint, "Skids: Masculine Hygiene," 2007. Courtesy of the artist.

Sound familiar? Quint's print ads feature Dean, age twenty-five, who knows "he can work hard, drink hard and play hard all weekend long without losing that 'extra fresh feeling,'" thanks to Skids; and Parker, age nineteen, who cycles with confidence with Skids in place. On her website, Quint makes explicit the point of the parody, inspired by her own analysis of conventional menstrual care ad campaigns over time: "The language, imagery and style are all in keeping with the tampon and maxi-pad adverts through the ages. Euphemism-laden, soft-focused and coy, these ads have influenced cultural taboos. . . . In light of this, we reckoned sometimes the only way to beat 'em is to join 'em."[56]

Radical Cheerleading

Still in the realm of irony, some radical menstruation activists engage in radical cheerleading—a reappropriative performance that troubles the boundary between disempowered and empowered femininity. Gaining a sneakered foothold in anarchist and punk communities and fast becoming a fixture at antiwar and antiglobalization protests, radical cheerleading reinvents a practice whose stereotype, at least, is emblematic of the worst of patriarchy.

In spring 2005 I observed a small group of Colorado State University student and community activists affiliated with the SEAC's national Tampaction campaign perform a series of cheers at the busy change of classes. One sporting a Mohawk and a bubble gum–pink net skirt, another festooned in a fuchsia feather boa and wearing hiking boots, they wove their way through the crowd shouting a cheer written for the occasion that introduces tampon alternatives and replaces "Hey Mickey" of Toni Brasil's pop hit with "Hey Tampon!"

Three sisters who decided to try out innovative forms of political protest founded the first squad of radical cheerleaders in 1996 and in 1997 published their cheer book (as a zine, naturally). Radical cheerleading spread rapidly and became a means to give voice to a wide range of social justice issues. According to Farrar and Warner, radical cheerleaders subvert gender norms through a spectacle of aggressive public display, rejection of cultural standards of propriety, and use of humor. This stylized form of street theater violates "the traditionally gendered practice of cheering to stage transgressive political spectacles that cannot easily be subsumed into or appropriated by mainstream political discourse."[57] Sparkle Motion, a Colorado-based radical cheer group, defines radical cheerleading as "activism with pom poms and middle fingers extended. It's screaming FUCK CAPITALISM while doing a split. . . . You don't have to be a dancer, coordinated, or even female-identified. . . . We're all about kicking corporate ass, taking on the social justice and women's issues of the day, and having a fucking blast doing it."[58]

Menstrual activists Brackin "Firecracker" Camp and Stiki Niki wrote "Blood Cheer" en route to a Southern Girls Convention (a grassroots gathering of anarcho-punk-identified women and girls).

Blood Cheer

(starts off to Beastie Boy Tune)

Let it go
Let your blood flow
Slow and low that is the tempo

I said . . . Let it go
Let your blood flow.
Slow and low that is the tempo

Hey ladies everywhere,
There's something you should know
About those products that you use
To plug up your flow

Those bleached tampons that you buy
Are full of dioxins
Instead of leaving your cunt cleansed
They leave it full of toxins

I say, let it go, let your blood flow
Slow and low that is the tempo
I say, let it go, let your blood flow
Slow and low that is the tempo

Hey grrls, everywhere
When you start your first blood flow
Don't be sad, instead be glad and let
That blood show

So smear it on your face
And rub it on your body
It's time to start
A menstrual party
You know it, I said
It's time to start a menstrual party

So let's howl at the moon
Repeat—howl at the moon
Let's get in tune (repeat)
To the cosmic rhythms (repeat)
Of our wombs (repeat)
So let's howl at the moon
(everyone howls)[59]

Camp performed the cheer decked out as a bloody tampon during a costume party at an all-woman Halloween celebration at a local Austin bar; she was the jubilant winner.

Although not a radical cheerleader, another activist uses performance in similar ways. Like EtShalom, who toured thirty-six cities, U.K.-based Chella Quint merges her skills as zinester and actor to spread the word about toxic conventional FemCare and healthier alternatives. Quint and her collaborator (and spouse), Sarah Thomasin took their Chart Your Cycle Roadshow through the northeast United States and more recently appeared at venues throughout the United Kingdom. The show includes readings from Quint's zines as solos and group sketches, and skits that feature "deconstructions of old feminine hygiene ads and attitudes using wit, irony and brute force." From advertising copy for Quint's appearance at the 2006 Newcastle Ladyfest: "It's part zine reading, part sketch comedy, part performance lecture. Highlights include: What it really feels like to use a mooncup, a leakage horror story you won't soon forget, and 1950s adverts performed before your very eyes![60]

Activist engagement with performance and street theater like Quint's and the radical cheerleaders on CSU's campus enjoy a rich tradition in the U.S. women's movement. Indeed, the coming-out party for the second wave of feminism began with performance. In August 1968 approximately a hundred members of the nascent women's liberation movement participated in a series of demonstrations at the Miss America pageant in Atlantic City, New Jersey. While the protest is mostly remembered for the Freedom Trash Can into which protestors tossed false eyelashes, wigs, girdles, curlers, and bras, other actions contributed to the "day-long boardwalk theater event."[61] A sheep was crowned Miss America and paraded down the boardwalk, and protestors performed a skit that depicted the miserable life of a typical American woman—tied to boring, low-wage work and tempted by the Revlon Lady, who promises to improve her life—urging her, "Get a whole new face, a whole new look, Buy Buy Buy."[62]

This kind of protest, often referred to as "zap action" (a form of guerrilla theater), proved an effective attention-getting strategy for the emerging second wave in its women's liberation movement wing. The short-lived group WITCH, the Womens International Terrorist Conspiracy from Hell, founded on Halloween 1968 by a small group of New York radical feminists, specialized in zap actions until the winter of 1969, when it redirected its focus to consciousness raising.[63] WITCH's first action was a hex of Wall Street (a choice I am sure today's radical menstruation activists would appreciate). Later, the coven descended on New York City and San Francisco bridal fairs, where WITCH chanted: "Here come the slaves. Off to their graves," a comment on the wedding ceremony as merely the transfer of woman as property. Other notable actions included Boston women hexing bars, Washington, D.C., women hexing President Richard Nixon's inauguration, and Chicago women hexing the chair of the University of Chicago Sociology Department, who had fired a popular woman professor.[64] One WITCH chant, chillingly resonant today, goes:

Double, bubble, war and rubble
When you mess with women, you'll be in trouble.
We're convicted of murder if abortion is planned.
Convicted of conspiracy if we fight for our rights
And burned at the stake when we stand up to fight.[65]

How different from such actions is a staged pep rally during which a small group of radical cheerleaders chant about the hazards of tampons and menstrual shame, or a series of skits mocking the FemCare industry?

Humor: Having Fun with Our Activism

Radical menstruation activists deploy a plethora of tactics to engage their audiences and to infuse an element of playfulness in their work, a value strongly associated with third-wave feminism. When Jennifer Baumgardner and Amy Richards, Reger, and others point out the ways third-wave feminists play with appearance, they are referring to play in the sense of experimentation or manipulation of makeup, hair, clothing, and piercings to please the self and send a message of agency. But radical menstrual activists' play takes a slightly different form (though they, too, are liberally pierced and dyed): They use humor to charm and disarm their audiences. Fully aware of the loaded nature of their content, they package the message in ways that can penetrate, sometimes slyly, the taboos that render menstrual talk off-limits. While the feminist-spiritualists tend to take themselves and the matter of menstruation very seriously, the radical menstruation wing can be heard a mile away, laughing out loud.

Campus-based menstrual activist Kristin Garvin, for example, says she describes herself "in a lot of crazy ways." Some of the labels she uses that "directly relate to my menstrual activism" include "radical eco-feminist, menstrual warrior, panty decorator, queen of periodia, empress of flow. . . . I like silly titles and think it's important to have fun with our activism."[66]

To loosen up the crowd at a menstrual health and politics workshop at Macalester College, one of the speakers invited those in attendance to discuss "the language of menstruation." She asked, "What are some of the most popular euphemisms used to name menstruation?" The usuals—"Aunt Flo," "the curse," and "on the rag"—were volunteered. The presenter, reading from an exhaustive list of euphemisms, A–Z, shared some of her favorites, including "massacre at the Y," and "arts and crafts week at panty camp." Some of my own favorites were "game day for the crimson tide," "Miss Scarlett's come home to Tara," and "Panty shield's up, Captain!"[67]

Some radical menstruation activists use cartoons to evoke laughter and critique simultaneously. A cartoon from activist Krissi Vanderberg's zine, *Crucial Sisterhood*, features Wonder Woman beating a cowering male physician with her speculum. Three other physicians lie at her feet, including one with a text by Freud near his head and another holding "prolife" literature. The caption reads: "With my speculum, I am strong! I can fight!" The mother of all menstrual activist zines at seventy-nine pages, *Femmenstruation Rites Rag* runs Karen Friedland's comic featuring Cunt Woman, a hand-drawn, crudely rendered image of a vulva with arms and hairy legs, who speaks in thought bubbles about such key topics as menarche, sex during menstruation, PMS, and tampon alternatives. Swedish activist Karolina Bång uses the playful medium of the comic strip to communicate rage. Her comic cum homage, "A Tribute to the Girl Who Actually Did It," rails against corporate ad campaigns too timid to reveal the true color of menstrual fluid, opting instead for an eerie blue substance of inexplicable origin. In-your-face humor that incorporates an element of shock to awaken consciousness is common in menstrual activist discourse. Such tactics run counter to the perception of feminists (of all eras) as humorless, dry, or overserious.[68] Their intent is to draw in readers who might otherwise find this taboo topic too gross or too personal.

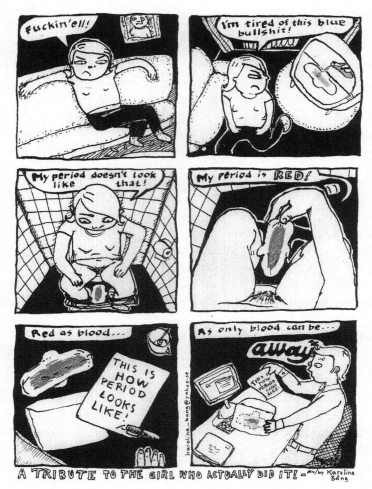

Figure 7. Karolina Bång, "A Tribute to the Girl Who Actually Did It," 2005. Courtesy of the artist.

Acting from a similar motivation are such women as artist and poet Geneva Kachman, who teamed up with filmmaker Molly Strange to found a holiday, Menstrual Monday, set on the Monday before Mother's Day. On the Menstrual Monday website (part of Kachman's online "Museum of the Menovultatory Lifetime"), Kachman and Strange explain the purpose of the holiday in the following way:

WHY? To create a sense of fun around menstruation; to encourage women to take charge of their menstrual and reproductive health care; to create greater visibility of menstruation, in film, print, music, and other media; and to enhance honesty about menstruation in our relationships.

How? Throw a *"Menstrual Monday party,"* any time of the year; hang Menstrual Drops and Splashes at your next Halloween event; organize a *"Sister Menses Costume Contest"*; view a Flofilm (a series of films with menstrual themes); invite your friends over for a messy spaghetti dinner; try some recipes that include ingredients from the Five Menstrual Monday Food Groups— green stuff, red stuff, chocolate, poppy seed, egg; hold a panel discussion on women's health issues; learn more about the Robin Danielson Tampon Safety Act (a federal bill that calls for independent testing of FemCare products, . . . mired in committee); flow-dye t-shirts; read menstrual-themed poetry–let your menstrutivity run wild! [69]

Kachman offers a bundle of creative party favors, including her menstrual drop and splash (a vertically twisted red pipe cleaner punctuated with a faux red jewel), ovum fans, PMS blow-outs, tamposes (roses fashioned from tampons), and my favorite, the UFO: Uterine Flying Object (a uterus fashioned of purple construction paper trailing long red satin ribbons representing menstrual fluid). Kachman's aim is transparent. A holiday supported by fun and funky accessories encourages participants to penetrate the taboo, get educated, and build community.

Sometimes radical menstruation humor is more subtle, relying on irony or reappropriation—taking images from one (typically sexist or trivial) context and imbuing them with new meaning in a different context—to capture attention and transform attitudes. The Bloodsisters are inventors of myriad graphics that liberally pepper their zines, brochures, workshop announcements, and website. For example, in their zine *Red Alert #2*, an image depicts vintage cowgirls, hips jutting as they grin provocatively, over the inscription: "Get Unplugged: Why Ride the Ol' Cotton Pony? Choose Reusables." Another image—grainy from the many times it has been reproduced—displays a model posing in her sleek 1950s-style block patterned bathing suit. Everything about her—the slightly arched back, sleek hair, high-fashion sunglasses, and stylish jewelry—exudes confidence, class, couture. The text beneath reads, "Our Revolution Has Style." Another image portrays "The Queen of Cups," a young woman sitting confidently on her wicker throne, surrounded by cats and Venus flytraps, in a t-shirt that reads "Hot" and a crown made of menstrual cups.

Another sly use of humor is at work in the making of menstrual product art, often in the form of outrageous headgear. On Walsh's website (www .Randomgirl.com), a menstrual cup makes another unlikely appearance: Illustrating her detailed discussion of alternative menstrual products, is a photograph of a grinning Donny Osmond doll wearing a Keeper as a hat. Some activists fashion crowns and tiaras from tampons, string, or glue and wear them in public spaces. Garvin, a.k.a. Queen Periodia, distributed instruction sheets on her campus at James Madison University that included directions for transforming oneself into "A Tampon Crown-Becoming Queen." A photograph of Garvin wearing her own tampon crown made it into the university's yearbook.[70] While making tampon headgear is a playful act, it is laced with the seriousness of direct confrontation. By bringing the instruments of standard FemCare out into the light of day and using them in unconventional ways—hats? tiaras? crowns?—it announces with a wink that we are not ashamed of our cycles. We are not afraid to handle—in public!—the products that we use to manage our flow. But on another level, by making art out of tampons—especially silly, frivolous crowns and tiaras—the activists thumb their noses at those very products and the industry that makes them. "This is what they're good for," they imply. "Don't put these toxic products in your body. They aren't healthy for you (or the planet)." This is parody in the service of social change.

When the social change is environmentally focused, tampon applicators are the target. At the time Canadian menstrual activists Liz Armstrong and Adrienne Scott launched the "Stop the Whitewash" campaign following the publication of their book by the same title, they commissioned environmentalist and artist Jay Critchley to fashion an ornate hat from discarded tampon applicators. Armstrong told me in an interview that this

> wonderful creation, which looked for all the world like a wedding cake (in three tiers, with a solar-powered propeller on top), never, ever failed to astonish and fascinate people (it disgusted a few too, but they were more disgusted when they realized that the applicators had been flushed down toilets and, especially during storms, had washed out by the thousands to sea, only to be tossed back on shore by ocean waves and tides). The hat started some incredible conversations and really got great discussions started on all sorts of issues related to menstrual taboos, menstrual health and environmental issues.[71]

The hat was even modeled by Bella Abzug, the fiery feminist politician known for her hats. Campaigners also constructed a giant menstrual pad with wings, large enough to be worn as a costume (with sunglasses and red sneakers), that read: "Always? Never." The costume appeared in many demonstrations, including one in front of P&G's Canadian headquarters in Toronto.

This was not the first time Critchley had worked with unconventional materials. In 1978 he began collecting nonbiodegradable plastic tampon applicators from Cape Cod beaches, the product, he said, of a dysfunctional Boston sewage system. He says he founded TACKI (Tampon Applicator Creative Klubs International) in 1985 to "further the creative use of these nonbiodegradable objects and ban their manufacture and sale through legislative action."[72] Critchley is perhaps best known for Miss Tampon Liberty, a gown he fashioned from three thousand found plastic tampon applicators, made in honor of the

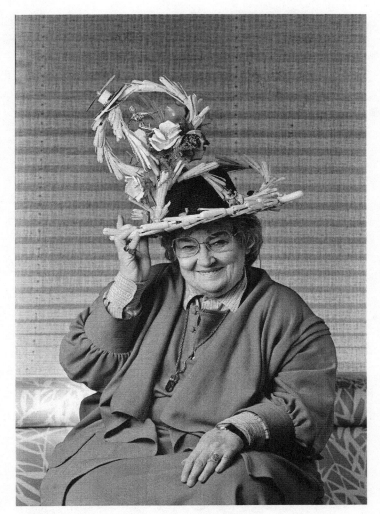

Figure 8. Bella Abzug modeling tampon applicator hat made by Jay Critchley, circa 1992. Photo © Chris McCallan.

centennial of the Statue of Liberty in 1986 and first worn at the Freedom for the Environment Rally at Liberty State Park. According to the artist, the gown is worn only on sacred occasions, such as appearances at the Massachusetts State House for legislative hearings. Miss Tampon Liberty came out of storage in 2000 when Critchley staged a performance piece titled "No with the Flow" to witness and lament the official turn-on of a 9.5-mile Boston sewage outfall pipe.

Humor characterized the products for sale by the Bloodsisters' small "alternative menstrual gear" DIY business, the now historic Urban Armour. From

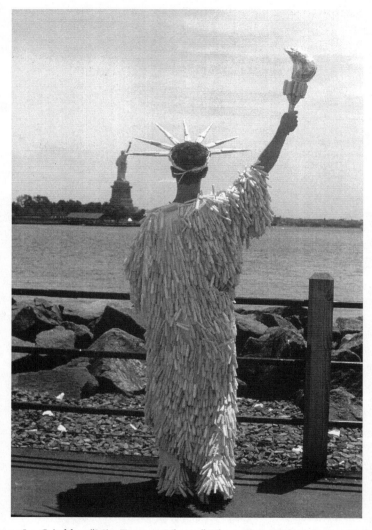

Figure 9. Jay Critchley, "Miss Tampon Liberty," Liberty State Park, 1989. Courtesy of the artist.

sales online and at Elle Corazon, a shop and community center in the Mile End neighborhood of Montreal, this modest venture supported their activist work. On the product line's website, the t-shirts, marketed as essential for surviving the perils of the urban scene, were introduced as "a clothing line created for the menstrual rebel, sporting emblems of the New Girl Power. . . . This is not fashion, this is protection." The t-shirts and panties sported silk-screened images that trouble assumptions and stereotypes, such as "Pussy Power," a winking cat (rumored to be an image associated with the sex-trade industry) wearing pearls.

Bloodsisters cofounder adee commented on the magnetic appeal of this reap-
propriated image: "More and more women are responding to the 'pussy power'
thing. And for us, pussy power is just a good place to begin—from there, you can
address even more issues about girl-body politics."[73]

Feminists have been laughing their way to social awareness for years. In her
introduction to *Pulling Our Own Strings*, a 1980 collection of feminist humor
and satire, Gloria Kaufman points out the long history of a feminist comic tradition. Beginning at least with the satiric classic *Lysistrata* (fifth century B.C.E.),
she argues, women have used humor to critique social conditions, disrupt the
dominant order, build woman-to-woman community, and release tension. She
also notes that "the suffrage movement created its share of platform wits—Anna
Howard Shaw, Sojourner Truth, Susan B. Anthony, Lucretia Mott, Harriet
Stanton Blatch, and Elizabeth Cady Stanton," as well as Marietta Holly and
Fanny Fern. The latter wrote "The Woman Question in 1872," a piece that artfully destroyed the popular antisuffrage claim that until women attained moder-
ation (in terms of clothing, spending and hairstyles), they were unfit for the
ballot. Kaufman admonishes her readers not to forget the contributions of past
feminist humorists because "their issues are today's issues. Although the tradition of feminist humor continued into the twentieth century, the current movement, which emerged in the 60s and has produced so much humor and satire of
its own, seems to have lost touch with the earlier feminist humor tradition."[74]

Certainly the now classic "If Men Could Menstruate," penned by Gloria
Steinem in 1977, is a wonderful example of menstruation-related humor that
packs a poignant punch. In spite of several dated pop-cultural references in the
piece (including fantasy menstrual products such as Joe Namath's Jock Shields
and Robert "Baretta" Blake Maxi Pads), readers, including my students, still
respond to the humor in this late 1970s piece. Here's an excerpt:

> What would happen, for instance, if suddenly, magically, men could menstru-
> ate and women could not? The answer is clear—menstruation would become
> an enviable, boast-worthy, masculine event: Men would brag about how long
> and how much. Boys would mark the onset of menses, that longed-for proof
> of manhood, with religious ritual and stag parties. Congress would fund a
> National Institute of Dysmenorrhea to help stamp out monthly discomforts.
> Sanitary supplies would be federally funded and free.[75]

Contemporary menstrual activists are indebted to this legacy of humor as they
produce their own lighthearted tools to stimulate dead-serious conversation and
promote personal and social change. Humor joins zines, e-zines, websites, and,
increasingly, blogs and various forms of social networking and performance to
constitute the radical menstruation activist toolkit. Indebted to its feminist past
and responsive to its current context, radical menstruation works to cultivate a

critical consciousness that challenges the power of the FemCare industry and urges menstruators to become their own agents of change. The route to change, they assert, is through DIY menstrual care, using needle and thread.

Stichin' 'n' Bitchin' for Change: DIY Menstrual Care

A mainstay of radical menstruation is DIY menstrual care. Once activists have spread awareness regarding the drawbacks of conventional FemCare, they then step in to offer the fix. Again, unlike earlier menstrual activists, they do not mobilize consumers to write letters to the FDA. And unlike the feminist-spiritualists, they do not stop at raising awareness. Their tactics are modest but subtly powerful, among them pad-making workshops whose leaders teach participants how to sew their own reusable cloth menstrual pads. These workshops, sometimes dubbed Stitch 'n' Bitch (popularized by *BUST* magazine founder Debbie Stoller, the label also refers to any needlecraft gathering) echo strategies used by second-wave radical feminists in the spirit of self-help. Typically combining information-sharing discussion and pad-making instruction, they reproduce the communal, body-centered approach pioneered by earlier feminist activists.[76]

I have attended many such events, including a particularly memorable workshop at tiny Macalester College in St. Paul, Minnesota, the outgrowth of a collaboration of the student environmental group E*Funk and the Community Service Office, among others. The event attracted thirty-some participants (including five men) plus one dog. After the participants heaped their plates with steaming brown rice, lentil stew, and green salad, the organizers presented the social, environmental, and health consequences of using conventional FemCare. Some visibly nervous, others more at ease, the team of presenters shared a passion for educating their peers about "the dirty little secrets" attached to mainstream care of the menstruating body.

At the close of the didactic portion of the workshop, the organizers invited the participants to work in small groups. First, we discussed a small collection of FemCare advertisements (for Seasonale, Tampax Pearl, and Playtex Gentle Glide) and short articles from popular magazines such as *Glamour* on menstrually themed topics. Then we responded to such probing questions as, "When was the first time you were exposed to menstruation?" and "How do you see menstruation portrayed in the media?" Last, we stitched brightly colored cloth menstrual pads (with wings!) under the patient guidance of the organizers, who circulated through the room. As we focused on our pads in progress, the room came alive with discussion. One man admitted that he hadn't understood before the workshop that the plastic or cardboard casing around a tampon was an applicator; he thought the whole apparatus was inserted in the body. The room erupted in laughter, including his own. A woman shared her realization that the applicators were designed to prevent self-touching.[77] In my own small group, we studied a string of alternative menstrual care products as they moved from group to group. Turning the Keeper over in his hand, a man half-joked that he'd "totally use it as a shot glass." In the midst of the discussion, the organizers glowed. This was precisely what they wanted: a robust turnout, a lively discussion, and a roomful of participants creating low-impact menstrual gear.[78]

Living the Legacy of Self-Help

Self-help, in the context of the women's health movement's emergence in the 1970s, shifted responsibility for wellness care from professionals to women themselves, transforming a deeply entrenched division of labor, notes medical sociologist Mary Zimmerman. In the 1970s, feminists formed self-help groups to meet their goals of women's empowerment; Zimmerman defines such groups as "any gathering of women who share common experiences, health care information and skills."[79] Typically small and similar in function and character to the feminist consciousness-raising groups that cropped up during the same era, second-wave self-help groups often focused on a specific health issue such as fertility or menopause. The expressed purpose of the groups was self-awareness through sharing information and experiences. The now famed Boston Women's Health Book Collective; Jane, the Chicago-based illegal abortion collective; and the Los Angeles Feminist Women's Health Center all began as feminist self-help groups.[80]

Zimmerman describes self-help as a process that effectively carries out three key objectives of the women's health movement. First, it is participatory and nonhierarchical, in opposition to the conventional doctor-patient relationship rooted in passivity and dominance. Second, it empowers women to become experts on their own bodies, a direct application of the premise that knowledge is power. And third, it favors noninterventionist, minimally invasive, and natural techniques for the treatment of illness, preferring, for example, nutrition, massage, and herbs to drugs and surgery.

Many of the underlying goals of the second-wave feminist health movement and its emphasis on self-help are present in menstrual activism, strengthened and updated by the DIY ethic. But today's target is different, and that's a key distinction. While the self-helpers of the women's health movement resisted what they experienced as an androcentric medical establishment, the radical menstruation activists identify the rise of global capitalism as the real enemy. While feminist health activists found fault with health-care professionals and positioned themselves in defiance to the medical establishment, the radical menstruation activists take issue with corporate entities that control menstrual discourse and, in their view, exploit negative menstrual attitudes to promote products the activists find dangerous to human bodies and the planet. This resistance is necessary, they believe, if we are to cure what one activist referred to as "the disease of capitalism."

COMPLEX CONNECTIONS AND DEPARTURES

This profile of the radical menstruation wing of the contemporary menstrual activism movement has revealed points of convergence and divergence with the feminist-spiritualists, the women's health activists who championed FemCare product safety in the 1970s and 1980s, and radical feminists more generally affiliated with the second-wave of the U.S. women's movement. The fractures, in particular, may lend insight into some of the debates at the heart of U.S. feminism today. Fundamentally, all menstrual activists, past and present, resist the sexism that undermines embodied agency. But the three groups of activists focus on different effects of this challenge. Early feminist activists contested the unsafe products that endangered women, working to reform the FemCare industry. Feminist-spiritualists, who have endured since the 1970s, challenge the de facto denigration of the menstrual cycle. Radical menstruation activists resist the corporate colonization of the menstruating body.

In the realm of tactics, both wings of the contemporary movement focus on everyday practices, but only the radical menstruation activists engage in a form of life politics that associates the personal with the global in the interest of social and cultural transformation beyond the self. Because the radical menstruation activists both critique the menstrual status quo and engage in radical structural change, I label their activism revolutionary. However, as these activists separate themselves from others in the menstrual activism movement, they fall in line with feminists of the previous generation when they "do feminism."

That is, the tactics they use to engage through disengagement are reminiscent of many radical feminist tactics practiced in the early second wave of the U.S. women's movement. Tracing from the present to the past, we see similarities that suggest an oft-neglected continuity between the waves. From zines to manifestos, radical cheerleading to zap actions, and DIY to self-help, all laced with a uniquely feminist brand of humor that persists over time, radical menstruation activists are generally unaware that they stand on the shoulders of the feminists who came before them. Many third-wavers, as I pointed out much earlier in the book, do not lovingly embrace their feminist history—indeed, many remain ignorant of it.[81] The history they do know compels them to righteously reject their mothers' feminism. U.S. second-wave feminism—admittedly imperfect— has been so devalued (and misunderstood) that today's feminists invest their energies in reinventing it in order to comfortably claim the identity "feminist."

In spite of the third wave's distancing from the second, parallels and continuities exist. Yet while some second-wavers refuse to acknowledge third-wave feminism as new, fresh, and innovative, this new form of feminism does distinguish itself in key ways, and we must pay attention to this reality as well. Feminism today is a social movement finding its balance between reliving its past and creating its future.

CHAPTER 6

Making Sense of
Movement Participation

When I first encountered the menstrual activism movement, I wasn't surprised when I scanned the human landscape. Almost immediately I detected something similar between the menstrual activists and the natural mothers, a variant of mother activists I studied several years ago. In fact, I am quite certain that my fascination with natural mothering led me—with almost magnetic force—to the Bloodsisters who introduced me to menstrual activism. During the mid-to-late 1990s I researched a loose network of mothers who embody a feminist critique of the denigration of women as mothers. Through alternative mothering practices, these women resist mainstream consumerism and the commodification of the body, the family, and the home. In my book that grew out of that research, *The Paradox of Natural Mothering*, I describe these natural mothers and interpret their back-to-basics, low-tech style of parenting as a paradoxical attempt at social change at the microlevel. While the mothers work to transform society one family at a time, they reify traditional gender norms rooted in essentialism and deference to nature.

There are definite connections between the menstrual activists and the natural mothers. Both movements embrace notions about bodies, health care, and consumerism that radically depart from the norm, enacting what Amy Richards and Jennifer Baumgardner call "everyday acts of defiance."[1] All thirty-two natural mothers I interviewed were white, almost all were college graduates (and many held advanced degrees), and most were married to men (and financially supported by their husbands' white-collar employment) and owned their own homes.[2] These data led me to argue that it takes privilege, or more precisely, Pierre Bourdieu's concept of "cultural capital," to adopt a lifestyle that violates dearly held and deeply entrenched cultural norms of parenting.[3] Natural mothering is high-risk activism. Breastfeeding a three-year-old in public, for example, can (and does) elicit negative responses. Choosing alternative health care over conventional options (such as refusing to treat a child's ear infection with anti-biotics) often meets resistance from mainstream health-care providers and even friends and family. So it made sense to me that the natural mothers are, for the most part, a privileged lot. Their privilege not only affords them access to the world of alternativity, but also protects them from the public censure that women with less cultural capital stand exposed to.

As I set about contacting and interviewing menstrual activists around the country, I wondered if a similar demographic profile would emerge, so I probed those I interviewed to reveal whom they saw as movement participants. One of the first interviews I conducted was with web-based menstrual activist Carol Church, who posted her (now defunct) e-zine *The Whirling Cervix* online. When I asked Church to describe "a typical menstrual activist," she offered the following: "I'd say that they tend to be environmentalists, feminists, matter-of-fact about sex and their bodies, and perhaps a little inclined to be the type who likes to shock people (not excluding myself here!)."[4] Based on the contacts I had made at that point through my fieldwork, I agreed with Church. I assumed that menstrual activists were risk takers and taboo smashers, women (and a few men) who felt bold enough to, as one activist put it, "make something private so public." Given this profile, the menstrual activists struck me as very similar to the natural mothers, so I expected to see white, middle-class, heterosexual women leading the charge to promote an alternative menstrual consciousness. And for the most part, I did.

But as I slowly accumulated demographic information from the activists I interviewed, a slightly different profile emerged. Most were white (88 percent), identified across the class spectrum (31 percent self-identified as working, poor, or lower class and 47 percent identified as middle class), and were college educated. Nearly all, as I expected, were women (94 percent).[5] But something surprised me: More than half the informants I had interviewed by the midpoint of my data collection identified as lesbian, gay, bisexual, transgender, or queer. Of those who fell into the LGBT category, most identified as queer. The second-largest number within this category chose an unconventional description of their sexual orientation, including "ambiguous," "undefined," and "no distinction." Several self-identified as "questioning."[6] Ultimately, 63 percent of the menstrual activists I interviewed identified as gay, lesbian, bisexual, queer, or in some way not heterosexual; hence-forth, I refer to these 63 percent as "queer." (Of the five women of color I inter-viewed, four fell into the "queer" category.)

What set of conditions could at once discourage a racially diverse movement and simultaneously encourage the participation of a large proportion of queers, themselves socially marginalized? The answer, I assert, is embedded in the rela-tionship each group has with sexuality. Women of color whose bodies have been constructed as "dirty," "animalistic," and "hypersexualized" as Patricia Hill Collins, bell hooks, and Dorothy Roberts, for example, have convincingly demonstrated, need a politics of respectability to secure cultural capital. Conversely, a politics of transgression shapes queer activist identity. In LGBT movements, challenges to what is culturally coded as transgressive are common, even central to movement activity. For queer activists, inhabiting a social and discursive location of outsider supports rather than impedes the risk-taking necessary to engage in menstrual activism, a form of resistance embedded in the menstrual taboo and its link to sexuality. Queer activists of color may be suspended between these poles and thus violate gendered race-specific norms when they do menstrual activism. Keeping in mind that four of the five menstrual activists of color I interviewed identified as queer, this tension is more than academic. One of these queer activists of color chose a pseudonym (only a very small number of the activists I interviewed did so) and another performs most of her activism in cyberspace. Could these choices reflect the challenges attached to the raced dimension of doing public activism around the body and taboo?

The Whiteness of Menstrual Activism

What might account for the overwhelming whiteness of the activists who challenge the menstrual status quo? Where are the activists of color? A number of explanations are possible. Is menstruation a low priority for women of color, engaged in a constant struggle for survival in a racist society? Relatedly, is the problematic social construction of menstruation merely a "luxury" issue—one that must wait in the wings while so many other issues press more aggressively for remedy? Or, taking a different tack, are the demographic realities of the movement little more than a microcosm of mainstream feminism and the issues that get the most attention? Perhaps personalized strategies of self-reliance, not public efforts at social change of the menstrual status quo, resonate more deeply for women of color. Here, I take up each of these possible explanations, exploring them in some depth.

Hierarchy of Needs?

When I interviewed a group of seven activists in Fort Collins, Colorado (a predominately white area of the United States), one young activist explained the lack of racial and ethnic diversity in the movement by comparing the historically white-dominated U.S. environmental movement with menstrual activism. Drawing on her college studies of the underrepresentation of people of color in the environmental movement, she argued that people of color were not engaged in some movements for social change because they were preoccupied with basic survival.[7] "Like first you need the basic things, like you need food and shelter and then it'll move up to these others things and on the top, then you can fight for justice or something and things that are not necessarily applicable to you. . . . Like the Hispanic activists and the Black activists and the gay activists focused inward on those issues, and then the white activists who don't have to necessarily focus inward on those issues, focus on other issues." Another activist in the room concurred: "People may not even be thinking about that or even have the time to, 'cause they have much other important, immediate concerns or values."

This "hierarchy of needs" explanation, though clearly in earnest, did not satisfy me. It seemed to assume, by effacing crucial differences between race and class, that all activists of color are necessarily lacking material privilege and thus struggling for basic survival. A more complicated rendering of identity that uses an intersectional analysis to make sense of an individual's (or a group's) social location resists such reduction. Thus the hierarchy of needs, itself a simple conflation of race and class, is inadequate to explain movement participation. Even if the logic of this explanation was not flawed, it would fail to explain the high representation of queers in the movement. The activist does not differentiate between activists of color and, as she puts it, "gay activists" when she lumps them all in the category of those whose basic survival needs are unmet and who are thus ill-equipped to engage menstrual activism.

Marginalization of Women of Color?

Sarah, a campus-based activist, offered this description of the demographic composition of the menstrual activism movement: "I think that menstrual activism ignores African American women. The leaders of the movement associate mostly with themselves, other white women. They dress and act really different than the African American women I know."[8] Notably and not untypically, Sarah's explanation focused exclusively on the whiteness of the movement (in spite of my question, which probed why the movement is overwhelmingly white and largely queer). When queried, few informants ventured an explanation for each of the demographic features I used to describe the movement. Most responses I gathered similarly focused exclusively on the raced dimension on the movement, and most informants narrowly defined "raced" as Black or African American, ignoring the absence of Latina, Asian, Native American, and bi/multiracial women. Given the vast differences among women of color, I resist extrapolating from explanations of the dearth of African American women in the menstrual activist movement to make sense of the absence of Latinas, Asians, and Native women, a quandary that calls for further research.[9]

I return to Sarah's point that the movement is trapped in a cycle of what Rosabeth Moss Kanter calls "homosocial reproduction." The movement is linked to and informed by the U.S. environmental and women's movements and heavily influenced by punk, all movements noted for their predominately white composition. For example, according to sociologist of punk culture Lauraine Leblanc: "While the contemporary punk subculture is largely non- or anti-racist, the origins of punk in the concerns of white British youth, the ongoing image of punks as racist, and the presence of other forms of stylistic resistance such as hip-hop function to exclude all but white youth."[10]

Many women of color, long aware of their lack of visibility in movements that claim to work for social justice, have called attention to the marginalization of their voices not only in the U.S. women's movement but also in key submovements, such as the reproductive rights/justice movement. For example, in a cluster of articles on reproductive justice in *NWSA Journal*, cluster editors Lynn Roberts, Loretta Ross, and M. Bahati Kuumba note the historic and persistent exclusivity of the U.S. women's movement: "White, middle class, mainstream—these are the monikers that are often used to describe the women's movement." By marginalizing the voices of women of color, they argue, the pro-choice movement (itself a raced framing of reproductive rights) has undermined its effectiveness to protect women's constitutional right to terminate their pregnancies.[11] Women of color have always been active in efforts to improve women's health, even if their efforts are not always acknowledged across race lines. Scholars have documented their crucial contributions to the fight for reproductive justice and HIV/AIDS, and numerous organizations have been formed by, for, and about women of color in the interest of health and wellness, such as the Black Women's Health Imperative (formerly the National Black Women's Health Project), the National Latina Health Network, the Asian-Pacific Resource and Research Centre for Women, and the Native American Women's Health Education Resource Center.[12]

But are women of color engaged in resisting the menstrual status quo? The negligible scholarly literature that examines U.S. women of color's menstrual and menopausal experiences almost exclusively focuses on Black/African American women and girls. Menstruation researchers acknowledge this neglect. McKeever's literature review of studies of menstrual shame, for example, explicitly notes the lack of ethnic representation among research subjects. Dorothy Hawthorne justifies her research into the symbols of menarche for recently menstruating African American girls based on the "paucity of literature describing menarche as a real-life event from the voices of African American females." Similarly, Shirley Dashiff states that "limited research exists on young girls' expectations of self care related to menarche. No studies specifically focus on Black girls"; her 1992 study of Black girls' self-agency attempts to address this lack. In their innovative study of rural African American women's responses to menopause, Elisha Nixon and colleagues note the "limited research on African American women's attitudes toward menopause."[13]

A few studies consider race in the context of menstrual and/or menopausal experiences: Clarissa Scott's research connects beliefs about the menstrual cycle and birth control; Woods, Dery and Most's research, which interrogates memories of menarche, current menstrual attitudes, and perimenstrual symptoms, included 33 percent African American women; and Janet Lee and Jennifer Sasser-Coen's interviews of women about menarche included 30 percent women of color, who variously identified as African American, Chicana, Mexican American, Asian American and Native American; the study, however, did not focus on the particular raced dimensions of menarcheal experiences.[14]

Menstruation Low on the Priority List?

If exploring menstrual attitudes and experiences of women and girls of color has not been a priority among researchers, could the same be said of women of color more generally, or at of least African American women? Opeyemi Parham, the African American physician turned holistic healer who offers workshops on "the blood mysteries" takes the following position: "Women of the African Diaspora do not prioritize this issue highly. That is because we don't have the luxury of time to think about this and because it is *too painful*" (emphasis Parham's). Parham may be right. A review of women's health websites geared to women of color does not reveal menstruation to be a major concern. For example, Women of Color Web, hosted by the Harvard University School of Public Health, posts articles regarding women of color and reproductive rights, birth control, sexualities, and feminism but includes nothing on menstruation.[15] The website Sistersong: Women of Color Reproductive Health Collective hosts no menstrually related content. The "Ask the Expert" column on the Black Women's Health Imperative website (formerly the National Black Women's Health Project), the only place menstruation and menopause appear on that site, addresses variability in menstrual cycle length along with menopause and weight gain. The websites of the National Latina Health Network, the Asian-Pacific Resource and Research Centre for Women, and the Native American Women's Health Education Resource Center host no menstruation-related content.[16]

Even health websites geared to girls of color (for whom the onset and early adjustment to menstruation is often a major concern) had minimal menstrual content: www.latinitasmagazine.com (geared to Latina girls), www.bamboogirl .com (geared to Asian American girls), and www.sistagirls.org (now defunct) include no mention of menstruation. Interestingly, sites that do not explicitly target girls of color tend to include at least some material on the menstrual cycle and its related issues. Gurl.com, which lists topics such as body image, DIY, health, sex, and "sucky emotions," includes a fair amount of menstrual content. Teenwire, an initiative of Planned Parenthood, goes so far as to include an animated tutorial for inserting tampons and even cups, as well as for applying pads. A multiracial young women's health site sponsored by Children's Hospital of Boston is the only site that includes a section on alternative menstrual products. Based on this limited information, it seems fair to conclude that, at least for now, there is a paucity of information that connects race/ethnicity and menstruation in both activist materials and contemporary academic literature.[17]

One reason menstruation is infrequently entertained as a legitimate issue for investigation and exploration may be the ways it has been framed in white dominant society. Amie "Breeze" Harper, the African American editor of the forthcoming anthology *Sistah Vegan! Food, Identity, Health, and Society: Black Female Vegans Speak*, is a burgeoning menstrual activist. Especially active in cyberspace, Harper writes and organizes in the interest of holistic health for women of the African diaspora, including the importance of practicing alternative femcare. When I interviewed her, Harper commented on the ways the menstrual activism movement is built upon "white racialized consciousness"—a concept she learned from the work of philosopher Arnold Farr and one she finds essential to understanding whiteness, white privilege, and the dynamics of raced inclusion and exclusion in social justice activism. Farr chooses "white racialized consciousness" or "the ways in which consciousness is shaped in terms of racist social structures" instead of "racism," which, he claims, "tends to imply that one has a conscious commitment to race-based discrimination." In response to my request to respond to the apparent whiteness of the menstrual activism movement, Harper wrote: "It has been my experience that when most whites involved in progressive social movement (such as holistic health, menstrual activism, alternative foods movements) fail to deeply engage with what their racialized consciousness means, do not understand how they potentially can and/or do embody white ontological beliefs even though they may not overtly embrace racism, prejudice or domination (especially domination that involves coercive control), can they fully recognize the ways their actions support and affirm the very structures of racist domination and oppression that they profess to see eradicated?"[18]

The whiteness of feeder movements such as holistic health (and punk and environmentalism, as mentioned earlier) not only influences the stream of individuals who embrace an alternative menstrual consciousness, but also shapes the movement itself, which typically reflects, as Harper states, "white ontological beliefs." Harper offered her own frustrated experience of white-dominated progressive social movements in which she, as one of the few Black women involved, understandably grows weary of the lack of racial awareness of movement participants, a lack that becomes an expectation that she, as a woman of color, can and should somehow correct. Generally speaking, without authentic engagement with the presence even of subtle racist structures and actions, movements are less than safe and affirming spaces for people of color. Women of color in white-dominated movements may experience tension, frustration, and annoyance at the ignorance and insensitivity of white movement participants who, for example, do not acknowledge the ways—both seen and unseen—that a white racialized consciousness constructs the movement.

This particular hegemonic consciousness produces a menstrual activist discourse that may not attract women who live daily with racism and classism. Harper points out that neither the approach to the issue nor the discourses used to articulate the movement's main message may appeal to women of color.

It could be that Black women who have never been exposed to menstrual activism could easily be persuaded to consider engaging in menstrual activism. Maybe it's simply the delivery, wording, or marketing that is *not working*; particularly if the delivery or educational models used are created by *white racialized consciousness.* What's more effective in dealing with working class women of color who are aware of the daily realities of racism and sexism on their bodies? Do we *first* approach them with how ecologically devastating menstrual products are? Or, do we create educational models in which anti-racism is at the core and connect menstrual activism to that? What is more appealing: present menstrual activism in literature that is "academic," or presenting it in music or oral narrative that first brings in the racism/classism struggles that Black women already have to deal with and then connecting it to *"decolonizing our reproductive gifts"*? Notice the language I used and who is the audience. *Menstrual activism vs. decolonizing our reproductive gifts.*[19]

If movement participants deployed the strategies and language Harper proposes, thus foregrounding struggles against oppression, they could create a context of understanding and engagement that resonates for socially marginalized women. This approach more appropriately sets the stage for discussions of and resistance to the commodification of the menstruating body than those conceived by white women who, due to their skin privilege, see primarily (or exclusively) the pain and struggle of their marginalized gender status.

Some women of color may resist mainstream menstrual culture by building their own movements underground or off the radar. When I asked Helynna Brooke, founder and owner of First Moon (makers of menarcheal celebration kits), to comment on the composition of the menstrual activism movement, she volunteered: "Most menstrual activists we have met have been white, middle class, although there is a quieter group of African American women who are working in their communities in a broader way than just focused on menstruation. Several African American friends have shared that their daughters have participated in yearlong coming-of-age programs that include a wide circle of women in the family."[20] The "broader way" Brooke references likely contextualizes menstruation in health-care activism or women and girls' empowerment. This is exciting work that I, in my extensive research, did not identify. Was I looking in the wrong places? Was I using the wrong language as I Googled, networked, and interviewed?[21]

My first exposure to menstrual activism was through the Bloodsisters, a collective of mostly white women in the context of the Michigan Womyn's Music Festival, an event that attracts a largely white following. From the beginning, my lens on the movement was white; I framed the issue in white terms expressed in white language and white tactics.[22] In other words, I found mostly white activists because, unwittingly, that's who I looked for. Sharon Powell, an African American health educator and artist who refers to herself as "the Coochie Lady," validated this hypothesis when I asked her in an e-mail interview if she could explain the particular demographics of the menstrual activism movement:

Perhaps [it is] due to the way [we] define activism and where we look for it. I have met some crunchy granola girls of color and of course, they are looked at as anomalies when they appear at conferences, in the college classroom, or at the lake. They might be accused of having white affectation or trying too hard to be multi-culti. On the other hand, there are women of color (and also men of color) talking about these things in other spheres. There is an African Holistic Health movement that has different ideas about the meaning of menstruation for women's health, particularly women of African descent. . . . Curanderismo [Southwest Mexican-American folk medicine] probably has things to say about periods, fertility, menopause. We do not call this activism. It is life . . . Members of All Red Nations [the women's organization of the American Indian Movement] have talked to me about their cultural practices around menstruation, fertility, et cetera.[23]

Powell touches on many issues here. First, she questions the definition of activism, challenging the artificial separation between doing activism and living life. Second, she suggests that menstrual activism is, at least in some cases, seen as a white thing. This may not only create difficulties for women of color who participate in the movement, but more fundamentally may serve as a disincentive to others from joining. Third, Powell acknowledges that there are movements such as African Holistic Health, practices like Mexican folk medicine, and communities such as Native American women activists that connect in some way with menstrual health practices.

My own white racial standpoint limited my data collection, blinding me to identifying practices and communities such as those described by Powell. This is a point I cannot overemphasize. Not only are the limits of snowball sampling laid bare, but more fundamentally, my own narrow definition of activism served as a barrier to a fuller, richer description of menstrual activism. Helyanna Brooke, who spoke of African American women who "work in their communities in a quieter way," Amie "Breeze" Harper, and Sharon Powell stimulated me to think beyond what was to me the obvious. Harper told of encountering the white-dominated holistic health, vegan, and alternative reproductive health movements and at first assuming that there were simply no Black people involved in these movements. After extensive web-based community building, including setting up her own website and discussion lists, she told me in a July 29, 2007, e-mail interview, she now realizes that

there is a big movement of people of color doing this in North America; it's just underground and doesn't seem to enter the Academy or mainstream literature. . . . I actually wonder if it's kept this way (protected) because there is fear of letting this "sacred" information "leak" into the mainstream movement (which is seen as white and anything "white or "euro-anglo" is suspicious). Much of the literature speaks of decolonizing the body and mind from white supremacy, whiteness, etc, I'm thinking that it's 'underground' because, 'Why would we let the "enemy" know about what we're doing to fight against systemic whiteness'?"

Harper's reflections reveal several possible explanations for the low numbers of women of color in the menstrual activism movement. Extrapolating from her observations and analysis of the larger alternative health movement of which menstrual activism is a part, we can imagine, first, that there *is* a parallel movement strategically protected from white mainstream society. Second, Harper's statement that "anything 'white' or 'euro-anglo' is suspicious" suggests that the framing of menstrual health and politics (as well as the strategies that derive from that framing) likely do not resonate for Black activists or other women of color. But at the same time that white racialized consciousness constructs a movement unaccommodating to women of color, it is possible that a Black or Asian or Latina or Native racialized consciousness (forged in response to and in defiance of white supremacist culture) renders public organizing around some aspects of women's health unappealing?

Staying Strong and Turning Inward

In a study of rural African American women's attitudes toward menopause, participants dealt with the menopausal transition by "staying strong." This is not a surprise, given the history of racism that has shaped the Black experience in the United States, including a long history of mistrust and suspicion of allopathic medical systems that have exploited members of Black communities (e.g., the infamous Tuskegee experiments).[24] In this study, menopausal African American women stayed strong either by turning inward and calling up their personal repertoire of resources (the preferred strategy), or they turned outward and pursued the support of others. The women resisted receiving help from others, especially doctors whom they did not trust. In fact, report Elisha Nixon and colleagues: "Turning to resources outside themselves was sometimes frowned upon as being counterproductive to staying strong because it threatened to disrupt their belief system and their reliance on spiritual faith, prayer and self efficacy."[25] These findings suggest another possible explanation for the absence of African American women (and perhaps of other women of color) in the menstrual activism movement. Individual-level solutions typically do not motivate social change. What would be the point of organizing women to take charge of their menstrual health when reaching outward and publicizing personal experience are stigmatized? For a woman who views faith and self-efficacy as the most productive means of self-care, organizing to increase health-care options, raising social awareness regarding the normalcy of the menopausal transition, or publicly challenging the medicalization of menopause would hold little appeal.

Thus, compelling explanations exist for the overrepresentation of whiteness in the menstrual activism movement I studied—the historic marginalization of women of color, their more pressing priorities, an inhospitable movement, and a Black women's ethic of strength and self-reliance. But many of these explanations come up short. And while we need to recognize the existence of a quieter, more underground menstrual activism framed in ways more sensitive to histories of racism, we must further explore what prevents these activists from bringing their work out into the daylight. In the section that follows, I turn to what might be at stake for women of color who breach certain culturally imposed standards, specifically for African American women who turn away from the "politics of sexual respectability."

THE POLITICS OF SEXUAL RESPECTABILITY

In *Righteous Discontent: The Women's Movement in the Black Baptist Church, 1880–1920*, Evelyn Brooks Higginbotham introduces the term "politics of respectability," a concept that asks each African American to "assume responsibility for behavioral self-regulation, and self-improvement along moral, educational and economic lines." She uses this term to characterize the Progressive-era activities of the Women's Convention of the Black Baptist Church. Championed especially by Black Baptist women, the "politics of respectability" dictated a life devoted to temperance, hygienic practices (of both the body and property), frugality, and self-representation that was mannerly and *sexually untainted*.[26]

Why a politics of respectability? Higginbotham argues that respectability was directed to two audiences: African Americans themselves and whites who, it was assumed, required "proof" that African Americans were worthy of respect. Higginbotham shows that African American women were particularly invested in promoting the standards of respectability, which, she argues, served a gatekeeping function, exacerbating class tensions between poor and more affluent African Americans.[27] Thus Black women social reformers, in a bid for earning the esteem of whites, engaged in surveillance—of themselves and of others—and marked class differences.

This project of asserting respectability responds to the historic social construction of the Black female body as promiscuous and sexually available. As Dorothy Roberts asserts in *Killing the Black Body*, the construction of the sexually voracious Black woman justified and continues to justify the denial of reproductive rights to Black women. To the assumption of Black female promiscuity, Hill Collins adds that

> images of working-class Black femininity that pivot on a Black woman's body politics of bitchiness, promiscuity, and abundant fertility also affect middle-class women. In essence, the controlling images associated with poor and working-class Black women become texts of what not to be. To achieve middle-class status, African American women must reject this gender-specific

version of authenticity in favor of a politics of respectability. They must figure out a way to become Black "ladies" by avoiding these working-class traps. Doing so means negotiating the complicated politics that accompany this triad of bitchiness, promiscuity, and fertility.

Just as Higginbotham showed how the politics of respectability reified class distinctions within Black communities in the late nineteenth and early twentieth centuries, Hill Collins demonstrates how contemporary notions of respectability operate to separate poor and working-class from middle-class Blacks today. Blacks who adopted so-called white values such as clean living and hard work fared best by white standards. These representations, embedded in what Hill Collins calls the "new racism," characterize Black people low on the social hierarchy as "untamed and in need of strict discipline.[28]

The tamed Black woman aspiring to middle-class status, then, is one whose sexuality is muted, even masked. Thus, a Black girl's entrance to womanhood is a crucial time to begin enforcing the rules of respectability. In Dorothy Hawthorne's study of African American mothers and their newly menstruating daughters, she found menarche was strongly linked with sexual availability. Simply put, when a girl begins her period, she is marked as ready for sex. In the interest of protecting girls' reputations, mothers, fathers, and grandparents caution the girls as they navigate their burgeoning sexuality. Some family members even hide their girl's menarcheal status. A powerful example of this practice (and its rationale) is captured in a story told to Hawthorne by a middle-class African American grandmother, remembering her husband's reaction at the time she announced their granddaughter's menarche:

> I told him [the child's grandfather] she had started. He said, "Woman, do you have to broadcast it? I don't want to hear nothing about it. I don't want to hear about it." That's him, I said. "Alright, okay." Then he said, "Don't you tell nobody else." That was that. You see your period, so you're ready for sex. That's what a lot of men think. So, I guess he doesn't want boys to think his [grand] daughter is ready or available for sex.[29]

Withholding this information, especially from boys, is an attempt to protect girls from sexual activity, because the sexually active girl cannot be the respectable girl.

Girls seem to quickly integrate the association between menstruation and sexual respectability. In subtle ways, they pass this knowledge girl to girl. Clarissa Scott and others' study of the emotional reactions to menarche of African American girls compared the results to an earlier study of white girls.[30] The researchers found no major attitudinal discrepancies between Black and white girls, but they did find rather dramatic differences in the messages the girls reported they would offer to a younger sister about her impending menstruation. While none of the white girls described menarche as a process of maturing,

27 percent of the Black girls did.[31] Clearly the meaning of menstruation differs across some racial categories; this difference, I hypothesize, is linked to difference between races in how bodies are represented, perceived, and acted on.

Of course, for all women and girls in Western culture, menstruation is constructed as a private matter, a personal issue typically deemed inappropriate for discussion either in public or with curious strangers conducting research. Layered with a legacy of the denigrated, hypersexualized body of color, the taboo for women of color may be even stronger than for white women. In Hawthorne's study of menarcheal African American girls and their mothers, twenty-one of the fifty-six volunteer mother-daughter pairs dropped out of the study because they viewed menstruation as "too private of a topic for open discussion."[32] (Would white mother-daughter pairs drop out at the same rate?) Consider this comment made in my October 18, 2006, e-mail interview of an anonymous African American informant, who proudly shared her journey to using alternative menstrual products: "I don't talk to women about my use of alternative products. When I first started using them I did and strangely people were disgusted by it. . . . Women I talked to who use tampons found the whole concept of inserting the Keeper as dirty or nasty. I experienced the same attitude in discussions of the pads even after I described how I soaked them, washed them in hot water and a little bleach and dried them. I know some Black women who had children who won't even use tampons because they think they are dirty."

Do Black women like these consider the products themselves dirty and nasty, or the body itself? Scott and others found that Blacks expressed feelings of revulsion regarding touching the vagina; Poland and Beane reported the belief among Black teenagers that the vagina is dirty.[33]

If the vagina is dirty, the respectable thing to do is to avoid it; to do otherwise violates norms of femininity. Accordingly, discussion of a bodily process particular to the female body is coded as inappropriate, unladylike talk. Proper ladies do not talk about dirty things. Harper echoed this sentiment when she wrote me in an e-mail: "Black women already have to deal with *proving* that we are 'ladies' (you know, 'on the same level and respect as white women'), so I guess if they engage in freeing their vaginas, maybe there could be a fear that they will make themselves appear 'unladylike.' I see so many Black women who straighten their hair to be 'more ladylike.' I'm wondering if avoiding dialogues with and researching information about menstrual activism makes them *think* they will jeopardize this."[34]

When I first talked with Parham on November 16, 2006, at the eighth annual Belly and Womb Conference and expressed my curiosity regarding the relative absence of women of color doing menstrual activist work, she smiled and referenced Black Baptist women as an example of a community especially invested in the politics of sexual respectability: "I fantasize about talking to a group of Black Baptist women. But it's just too risky. Our sexuality has been used against us. We are leery of going 'down there.'" "Down there" is loaded for women of color, not only the site of pleasure and for some, procreation, but also a site historically exploited. "Down there" is painful and dangerous. For Parham, Black women's detachment from their bodies is the consequence of a torturous string of events Black women have endured throughout a history that reaches back to certain patriarchal practices and extends through slavery and institutional racism.

> First we were betrayed by our men, who created female genital mutilation, in our West African homes. Next, we were betrayed by our race, as other Black people sold us into slavery to white people. Then, we were betrayed by our adopted culture as the "First World" redefined us as less than human, without spirit, and bestial. Yes, this last was true for Black men, also, but it is especially true for Black women. To this day, we hold a reactive, protective emptiness inside, where we should carry creativity, power, lust and passion. All these things can (sometimes) come from the heart, but NEVER the groin. So . . . you won't see many Black women tasting their own menstrual blood.[35]

PUTTING MARGINALIZATION TO WORK

While most menstrual activists are not likely to taste their menstrual blood, a sizeable number engage the menstruating body in a context quite different than do straight women of color. When I asked Matt Reitman, a campus-based menstrual activist, to comment on the demographic profile of the movement, he responded with confidence and ease. From the vantage point of someone who self-identifies as "nonheterosexual," the "queerness" of the movement was obvious: "[The movement] is queer because sex and sexuality-related issues are already acceptable and expected in queer communities, so it is a relatively easy campaign to pitch to this group."[36]

For Reitman, sexuality's central place in queer communities predisposes their members to engage with menstruation, an embodied process connected to sexuality. At the same time, queer stigmatization is inextricably linked to gender identity. In the context of a heteronormative culture that codes homosexuality as a transgression against gender norms, being queer is a challenge to notions about femininity and masculinity. Because heterosexuality is in this culture a cornerstone of legitimate gendered identity, those who resist the heterosexual mandate are suspect, coded as deviants, outsiders, freaks. In the words of queer theorist Michael Warner:

> Every person who comes to a queer self-understanding knows in one way or another that her stigmatization is connected with gender, the family, notions of individual freedom, the state, public speech, consumption and desire, nature and culture, maturation, reproductive politics, racial and national fantasy, class identity, truth and trust, censorship, intimate life and social display,

terror and violence, health care, and deep cultural norms about the bearing of the body. Being queer means fighting about these issues all the time, locally and piecemeal but always with consequences. It means being able, more or less articulately, to challenge the common understanding of what gender difference means, or what the state is for, *or what "health" entails*, or what would define fairness, *or what a good relation to the planet's environment would be.*

Here, Warner explicitly articulates queer identity as a platform for a progressive social consciousness, pointing in particular to queer's radical potential to question "deep cultural norms about the bearing of the body." While living on the margins is precarious, often dangerous (even lethal), for queers, it can, in some contexts, serve as a site of personal and political agency, especially for those emboldened by race and class privileges, such as white queers and middle-class queers. As Josh Gamson reminds us, the "fixed" identity queer, like other identity movements (racial, ethnic, gender), can serve at once as a basis for oppression and political power. However ironic it is to see queerness as fixed when it is itself a statement of fluidity, the point is clear: In some cases, claiming and living a queer life may facilitate certain resistances. Michael Warner echoes this point: "Queer politics opposes society itself."[37]

As Sheri Winston, holistic health and sexuality educator (who self-identifies as "98 percent heterosexual"), reasoned in our interview: "I think in that at least the people I know who are, or fall in [the queer] category, it's because they are already so radical. They're already so outside so there's an advantage to being the outsider."[38] Here Winston asserts that individuals who are radical exist on the social margins, a vantage point from which they can see what those on the inside may not, and thus do what they may be too timid (or perhaps more prudent, given the potential consequences) to do. If the queer life inspires, even demands, reflection on and critique of hegemonic discourses and practices, then queers are well positioned to extend their critique to any number of social norms, including the menstrual status quo. Already widely regarded as gender benders through the lens of heteronormativity, queers may in some cases be freer to play with gender norms. Perhaps this was openly lesbian filmmaker Barbara Hammer's thinking when in 1974 she created the path-breaking short *Menses*, mentioned earlier. As one of the Fort Collins activists noted in reference to public menstrual talk: "It's just not very, I think, appropriate within the confines of what's considered female to talk about something that's considered gross and [im]polite." If an individual exists outside the "confines of what's considered female," perhaps it is a bit easier to shatter the polite silence surrounding menstruation. I do not mean to suggest, however, that queer identity necessarily makes high-risk activism, such as menstrual activism, easy, or as Reitman implies, "natural."

I do not suggest that all or even most queers are interested in doing this work (or are compelled to entertain a critique of normative menstrual culture). I am suggesting for queer-identified activists who are already putting their bodies on the line, engagement with menstrual activism may not be as significant (although no less perilous) a leap as it might be for individuals invested in and rewarded for playing by the rules.

Indeed, the risk taking and taboo smashing at the center of menstrual activism may be for some activists a rich reward for doing the hard work of social activism. And given that most of the queer-identified menstrual activists were white, their race privilege may enable them to go public with the private, without risking the racist censure that disciplines the body of color. This is the case for campus-based Rachel Warner (who identifies as "queer/dyke"), whom I asked what she found especially rewarding about being a menstrual activist: "I like being able to talk about a taboo subject and in doing so work on breaking the taboo." While I found that queer-identified menstrual activists often cited the thrill of transgressing social boundaries as a benefit of the work, I did not hear this from queers of color active in the movement, affirming Gamson's contention that "queer does not so much rebel against outsider status but revel in it." Could the tension between the politics of respectability and the politics of transgression mute the activism of queer women of color?[39]

In fact, many of the higher-risk, more public strategies menstrual activists used were the work of white, queer-identified movement participants. Activists who produced the boldest zines with the most outrageous language and graphic imagery, including the creator of the cartoon "Cunt Woman," and more than half the radical cheerleaders publicly identify as queer, lesbian, bisexual, or in some cases "not heterosexual," "undefined," or "somewhere between homo and hetero." I am not suggesting a hierarchy of activism here that equates bold with better or more effective; in fact, some would argue that the more outrageous menstrual activism is less effective because it tends to offend and shock. But I am suggesting that the risks attached to the in-your-face tactics of menstrual activism might be too great for women subjected to the racist gaze.

Many movement leaders, including former student coordinators for the Student Environmental Action Coalition's Tampaction campaign, a founder of the Bloodsisters, the organizer of the first Anti Tampon conference, the founder of the online Vulva Museum, the founder of POW—Pissed Off Women (who produced the widely circulated mock Tampax ads discussed in chapter 5)—and the leader of the successful anti-chlorine-bleaching campaign in the United Kingdom—all, due to their sexual orientation (which they publicly identified), are sexual outsiders. For example, the cover of the fourth issue of queer-identified Chella Quint's zine *Adventures in Menstruating* features a rear shot of two women in wedding gowns, holding hands—Quint and her "gaywife" (a term she created to keep the queer in lesbian marriage). Quint's reasons for choosing this image are complex and interrelated. She wanted to put "a lesbian wedding on display in people's homes, in bookstores, in libraries, in cafés, and on the

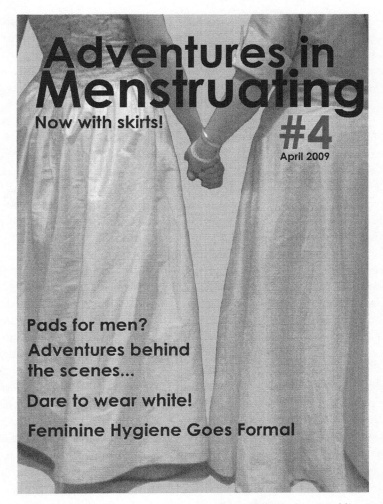

Figure 10. Chella Quint, *Adventures in Menstruating* #4 ("The Lesbian Wedding Issue"), cover, 2009. Courtesy of the artist.

Internet, and . . . say a big 'fuck you' to Prop Eight." And she chose the wedding dresses to culture jam a Tampax ad campaign running in the U.K; with the tagline "Now with Skirts!" she references the Tampax Plus Skirt (a tampon topped with a small fan of cotton wadding designed to catch fluid before it leaks). The advertising campaign, says Quint, features "miniskirts and scantily-clad women." In the zine, she takes the campaign to task along with other "freakishly formalwear themed 'innovations' that have come out recently." Here, Quint turns up the volume of her message by pairing queer with a talk-back to commercial FemCare.[40]

If transgressing boundaries is, in Reitman's words, "already accepted and expected" in queer communities, it makes sense that the menstrual activism movement, itself rooted in transgression, would serve as a gateway of sorts for high numbers of queer activists. In contrast, the politics of sexual respectability may serve as a barrier to African American women's access to the movement (and possibly to other women of color as well). While Black women, for instance, struggle to be seen as proper ladies, women already deemed unladylike (and men deemed unmanly) because of their sexual orientation may experience more freedom to push back against the boundaries that define them as deviant.

The queer body that, in the context of heteronormative culture, exists in the realm of the disrespected and marginalized can, under some conditions, exploit this subject location. The small group of Fort Collins–based radical cheerleaders I observed in spring 2005, for example, one bald and another sporting a small Mohawk, in their funky cheerleading costumes rhythmically shouted about tampons, pads, cups, and sponges in the center of their large university campus. Some passersby shook their heads, smiling; others' jaws dropped in amazement. Their comments ranged widely, from "Are they talking about what I think they are talking about?" to "Is nothing sacred?" to "Now I've seen everything!" But one comment that perhaps more than anything suggests that the politics of transgression is intimately linked to doing menstrual activism came from a young woman who turned to her male companion and exclaimed with disgust: "I can't believe they are talking about tampons on the plaza. But what do you expect from a bunch of lezzies? It figures." Her assumption that so-called deviant sexuality (read into the cheerleaders' unconventional, gender-bending presentation) presupposes rebellion in more general terms (i.e., of course a lesbian would make an issue of menstruation) lays bare the link between deviant identity and deviant attitudes and actions.

Yet the formulation I advance—queer as a site of resistance—too easily reifies what political scientist Cathy Cohen calls a "queer-straight divide" that privileges homosexuality as the main (or only) characteristic that shapes marginalization and obscures the complexity of identity. In describing queers as socially marginalized, I am not suggesting that the lack of sexuality privilege definitely or completely constructs queer individuals as disadvantaged; not all queers are created equal. Race, gender, class, physical ability, citizen status, and myriad other axes of identity shape the distribution of privilege. Cohen asserts that the "radical potential of queer" in fact lies in dismantling the queer-straight binary, which itself grows out of a privileged standpoint and fails to adequately analyze what she calls the "marginalized relation to power."[41] Still, given the strength and persistence of heteronormativity that constructs lesbians, gays, and bisexuals as sexual deviants, I find it useful and important to ask why queers, as individuals who lack some measure of privilege and are often exposed to public censure and invalidation, would find their way to a movement that requires high-risk participation.

What forces simultaneously repel those marginalized by racism and attract those marginalized by sexuality, and how can we make sense of the participation of those who fit both categories? I began with that question and ended with dozens, among them, Might I be chasing the wrong line of inquiry? Might a more fruitful set of questions lead me to ask how my research methods emerged from my particular social location and my limited framing of menstrual activism, as theory and praxis? And if the demographic profile I identified is a distortion—a partial picture of the movement as seen through the myopia of white racialized consciousness—how do I ascertain the true diversity of menstrual activism? Or perhaps the profile I uncovered is not a fiction but more precisely a reflection of authentic racial differences that approach the culturally freighted issue of menstruation in myriad ways. For instance, could the menstrual taboo be low on the priority list of activist issues, or at least be managed in the sphere of the private and at the level of the individual for some communities of color? Or might the politics of respectability that Higginbotham found central to the identity of Black Baptist women in the late nineteenth and early twentieth centuries, as I posit, remain a barrier to engagement with the menstrual taboo for activists of color? If the politics of respectability is a factor that regulates movement participation, could the reverse of this standard—a politics of sexual transgression—inspire some of those marginalized by their identity as sexual outsiders to breach boundaries and rewrite the rules of the body and its care? And how can any of these questions be responsibly answered without effacing the complexities of identity that reify a queer-straight divide or conflating raced experiences into the indiscriminate and unwieldy notion of "women of color"? Finally, how can any explanation for the whiteness and queerness of the menstrual activism movement—however tenuous that characterization may be— take into full account the presence (and absence) of queer activists of color? While I can hardly settle these questions, I can hope to enliven them with the textures and nuances unique to empirical study. Here, the questions become real and the answers, I hope, within our grasp. Through the menstrual activists, we can glimpse the constellation of factors that both facilitate and impede political action while shedding light on the politics of identity that shape not only social movement participation, but also the very research processes engaged in the quest for understanding.

CHAPTER 7

When "Women" Becomes
"Menstruators"

The sum of our small rebellions combined will destabilize the normative gender system as we know it.

—Emi Koyama, "The Transfeminist Manifesto"

It seems that feminism is in a mess, unable to stabilize the terms that facilitate a meaningful agenda.

—Judith Butler, *Undoing Gender*

A Korean FemCare commercial begins with a long shot of a beautiful woman striking a provocative yet demure pose in a navy blue, form-fitting dress, seated on the edge of a chair in front of a circular window that looks out on the lush green outdoors. Our eye is drawn to her long, slender legs, crossed at the ankles. We hear strains of ethereal music—a harp and a solo soprano. A succession of close-up shots follows. Frame by frame, the woman wordlessly communicates confidence, sensuality, innocence, and playfulness, all with the utmost femininity, as a woman's voiceover almost whispers: "There is something that I really want to do. . . . Jealousy?" (The woman looks down and smiles coyly.) "Love?" As the commercial cuts to a graphic of a disposable menstrual pad, the voiceover continues: "News of the day that will be remembered with herb scent." The music shifts abruptly to a chorus of cellos, which rapidly play three deep tones, sustaining the last. We see an extreme close-up of the large window, which now resembles an illuminated moon. The camera settles on the woman's model-perfect profile, her long black hair blowing in the wind. She turns to the camera and as her mouth settles into a smug smile, her head cocked, the voiceover concludes: "UFT . . . Because I am woman."[1]

A beautiful woman, the symbolism of the moon, a product innovation—these are unremarkable in a FemCare commercial. But this is far from a typical commercial for menstrual pads. The advertisers assume that Korean viewers will read the subtext of the commercial's final statement, "Because I am woman," paired with the woman's smug (or is it triumphant?) smile. Indeed, UFT, a Taiwanese FemCare company, is no doubt banking on the subtext to sell product, for the star of this commercial is Harisu, a celebrated Korean model/pop singer and actress known widely as a postoperative male to female transsexual.[2]

In 2004 at the time of this commercial, Harisu was all the rage in Korea; her single "Foxy Lady" was at the top of the charts. UFT hired Harisu—the first transgender individual to appear in an ad for FemCare products of any kind—to launch its campaign promoting a new line of menstrual pads. Although at first Harisu declined, when she learned that the herb-enhanced pads promise to reduce menstrual cramps, she accepted the offer.[3] Optimistically speaking, Harisu's appearance in this context could signal a climate of increasing acceptance of transpersons, or at least UFT's assumption that consumers would read their choice as a reflection of their progressive values. Or it could portend something subtler but strikingly profound: the changing relative salience of gender to sex and the potential of identity detached from embodiment.[4]

UFT's commercial and its unconventional star represent an acute unresolved conceptual tension within both the menstrual activism movement and feminist politics more generally: What should feminists do about the category "woman"? Feminist theorists generally agree that perceptions of biological difference are the basis of the bifurcated gender paradigm expressed through oppositional categories—male and female, woman and man, masculine and feminine. But theorists differ when it comes to what to do about that paradigm: work within it or destroy it?

Gender theorists see gender as a status achieved in and through interaction and seek to dismantle systems of domination and subordination by interrogating, to quote Johanna Foster, "the construction, deployment, and reification of a multiplicity of identity categories as social practice."[5] Alternatively, sexual difference theorists see gender as an attribute possessed by individuals and advocate affirmation of the feminine as political strategy.[6] In other words, sexual difference theorists embrace the category "woman" and work to recuperate it through the explicit valuation of women qua women. Gender theorists, on the other hand, wish to smash the category itself. But worries linger even among the gender theorists who march under the radical banner: If feminism is grounded in the lived experience of women's bodies, what happens when the body disappears? Because menstruation exists at the complicated crossroad between sex and gender, it sheds a unique light on this recurrent dilemma in feminist thought. Menstrual activism—fixated on messy, bloody bodies—provides us with a rich opportunity to explore what happens when we detach woman from body and what happens when we don't.

While feminist-spiritualists (most aligned with sexual difference theory) rely on the category "woman" as a basis for political action, radical menstruation activists (most aligned with gender theory), inspired by third-wave feminism, reject the category "woman."[7] Through a campaign of transinclusion, they make gender trouble by "queering" menstruation when they refer not to women who menstruate but to "menstruators." This strategic language serves a pedagogical function: it models a concrete dismantling of the gendered social order and demonstrates that when the body is detached from identity, feminism does not wither away; rather, we can mobilize around the experiential. Linda Alcoff in her classic 1986 essay "Cultural Feminism versus Post-Structuralism: The Identity Crisis in Feminist Theory" pushed for a conception of subject as positional in which a woman is defined not by *who* (or by her attributes) but by *where* (or by her context): "The concept of positionality allows for a determinate fluidity of woman that does not fall into essentialism; woman is a position from which a feminist politics can emerge."[8]

But radical menstruation does more: It helps us put theorizing like Alcoff's to work and illustrates—in real terms—how we can challenge sexism without reifying a fundamentally flawed category. The radical menstruation tactic of referring to "menstruators" (instead of "women") as an acknowledgement of the sexed dimension of menstruation—a bodily process that exists not independently of, but in relationship to, the gendered body—is a progressive development. Speaking of "menstruators" signals a genuinely inclusive menstrual discourse that with each utterance challenges an essentialist gender binary. While the feminist-spiritualist approach, foregrounding the salience of gender identification, also contributes something worthwhile, its frame is limited by a false assumption of the unity of women, based on an essentialist conception of womanhood implicitly defined as white and middle class (see chapter 4). Third-wave feminism, as expressed through radical menstruation activism, demonstrates that fixed identities, acknowledged as imperfect and limiting but politically expedient, can and should be destabilized in the interest of social justice. This linguistic choice (and its practical implications) serves as the most compelling evidence that third-wave feminism represents a transformation under way in the U.S. women's movement.

WOMEN, BODIES, MENSTRUATION: WHAT'S IN A CATEGORY?

As long as menstruation is attached to the sexed body (that is, generally speaking, *females* menstruate), the experience of menstruation is coded as women's experience, as Harisu, as the hyperfeminine transsexual spokesperson for menstrual pads, illustrates.[9] Born a male, Harisu lacks the biological capacity to menstruate, yet her gender presentation of a hyperfeminine woman contradicts this material reality. Important to the consumer, the corporate executives who recruited her assume, is the association of menstruation with femininity, or with womanhood more generally. And no one could outdo Harisu as representative of classic femininity. At the same time, UFT's choice of a transwoman exploits the ambiguity attached to bodies at once biologically male and undeniably female. That is, Harisu as menstrual spokesperson implies a bending, if not a breaking, of the rules of who speaks for menstruation. Furthermore, positioning Harisu as a spokesperson for a FemCare product lays bare (literally, perhaps) palpable tensions between the feminist-spiritualist and the radical menstruation approaches to social change.

These tensions, when interrogated, concretize what's at stake in a debate at the heart of feminist theory—the tug-of-war between those who embrace sexual difference theory and those who embrace gender theory as the conceptual fodder for feminist politics. Interestingly, the two wings of the movement are relatively isolated from each other. During my fieldwork, I encountered radical menstruation activists who, often through characterization, derided feminist spiritualism. For example, one activist's shorthand for feminist-spiritualists is "hippie-dippie-moon-love." Radical menstruation activists, on the other hand, seem relatively off the radar of the feminist-spiritualists. When the feminist-spiritualists did mention their movement counterparts, (usually in response to my direct inquiries), their responses were inflected with mild bemusement, though typically not disparagement.

In the history of menstrual activism, the move to gender neutralize menstruation is relatively recent. In the mid-1980s, for instance, when members of the Boston Women's Health Book Collective (BWHBC) initiated letter-writing campaigns to pressure FDA officials to mandate standardized tampon absorbency ratings, they appealed to those on their mass mailing list with the salutation (not surprisingly) "Dear Women."[10]

"Work It Girl!" or Taking Offense?

When I stumbled upon Harisu's appearance in UFT's ads, I was, of course, fascinated by the implications of a transsexual selling, in the parlance of the transgender community, a "biowoman's" product.[11] *PersuAsian*, self-described as "a newsmagazine for the gay Asian and Pacific Islander Men of New York," reprinted the story of Harisu as UFT spokesperson adding only the comment: "Work it girl!—Eds."[12] Another web-based news site, transgenderonline, names Harisu one of the "Transgender People of the Month" (January 2006), ostensibly for her commitment to transgender visibility.

But how would contemporary menstrual activists respond to UFT's commercial starring Harisu? Many feminist-spiritualists, I venture, would be greatly troubled to find Harisu the spokesperson for a line of menstrual products. I would expect a rush of indignant questions: What does *she* know about menstruation? Is UFT trying to take menstruation away from women? Isn't this another example of the cultural disregard for the uniqueness of womanhood and the sacredness of menstruation? Positioning a transsexual woman at the center of a FemCare campaign, they might argue, reduces menstruation to little more than a commodity. Disrespect for the biological process (and more generally, for women) is a sore spot for these activists. Rooted in a cultural feminist sensibility that fortifies the category "woman," they see menstruation as a sacred, honorable, and unique gift of womanhood.

Alternatively, many associated with the radical menstruation wing of the movement would likely view with ambivalence Harisu as a menstrual product spokesperson. While they would agree that the commodification of menstruation is egregious and must be defied (keeping in mind their posture of corporate resistance), I suspect they would also celebrate the choice of a transsexual to front menstrual products. Not only would the activists be thrilled that Harisu's identity as a woman must be taken seriously for the commercial to work, but also they would applaud the ad as a political statement that implicitly acknowledges that authority over menstruation is not limited to biological women.

"We're Making Bleedin' Everyone's Issue"

In her zine *Red Scare #3*, Fawn P. struggles in her introductory essay with menstrual activism that discursively fails to include transpersons: "I've been working on menstruation-related stuff for quite a while now, and there's an element of it that makes me uncomfortable." Referencing the undeniably controversial "womyn-born womyn" policy of the Michigan Womyn's Music Festival, she asks: "Why shut an M to F trannie out of your music festival (or a transitioning F to M)? Just to reduce things to this minimum, to set up a fence, to establish a false qualifier for all those who are allowed in? It's like only letting the 'real' Americans run for president, or only letting the 'real' couples get married in your church. I wonder if this isn't what we're doing with menstrual activism sometimes. It's true, we all come from cunt, but we don't all bleed, and menstruation isn't the thing that makes us all 'womyn.'"[13]

In a similar vein, Marie Abbondanza produced an insert for her zine *It's Your Fucking Body: Reclaim Your Cunt* that details her realization regarding radical menstruation:

> i've realized over the past few weeks that all of the resources I've come across concerning radical menstruation (including the ones I have written) seem to neglect these 2 really important facts:
>
> 1. NOT ALL WOMEN MENSTRUATE
> 2. NOT JUST WOMEN MENSTRUATE
>
> Blanket statements that seem to be really prevalent within this movement like "all women menstruate" I think are supposed to "bring us together" but do just the opposite. Statements like that completely invalidate transwomen and non-trans women who do not bleed for a variety of reasons. Not all women

menstruate. Lots of non-trans women don't menstruate due to different diseases, cancers, surgical procedures, and just plain menopause and hysterectomy, although transwomen maybe don't have the same need for this information, it's still really crappy to exclude them from our definition of WOMAN by basing it completely on a physical function that some of us experience and some us don't. [14]

Here Abbondanza articulates the need to include as "women" not only transgendered people and transsexuals, but also any biological woman who, for any number of reasons, does not menstruate. That is, she argues for a generally expansive movement rooted in a nonbiological definition of "woman" (or perhaps no definition at all). When she acknowledges that some individuals may not want or need menstrual information, her point is less about building a diverse movement, per se, than about articulating an inclusiveness that erodes barriers based on biological realities.

The Student Environmental Actions Coalition (SEAC)'s Tampaction campaign took this view one step further by making intentional linguistic choices in its materials: They refer to one who menstruates not as "woman" but as "menstruator": "We say 'menstrual health' instead of women's health because this is an issue of menstruation, not of gender. Not all women menstruate, not all people who menstruate are women. We're letting the world know that bleedin' can be everyone's issue."[15] SEAC's push to degender menstruation was directed by Yonah EtShalom when squee coordinated the Tampaction campaign. (EtShalom, as mentioned earlier, devised the gender-neutral pronouns "squee" and "squir," and identifies as "genderqueer.") Subsequent coordinators have continued this work, and EtShalom has continued to prioritize transinclusion in menstrual activist work since leaving squir SEAC post, choosing to name squir resource center Below the Belt: A Resource Center on Genital, Sexual, and Reproductive Health. EtShalom avoids gender specificity in phrases like "women's health." For EtShalom, services and information should be directed to people who need them, whatever their gender expression. On squir website, EtShalom includes an extended explanation of who menstruates and who does not, in the process making clear the importance of gender-neutral language in the context of menstrual discourse:

who menstruates?

Lots of people menstruate. Lots of people don't. Contrary to wide teachings and misconceptions, not all wimmin menstruate and not all menstruators are wimmin.

For example:

Menstruators who are not wimmin are people who have vaginas and uteruses, but do not call themselves wimmin. They have been born with these

sex organs but they don't identify with the term "wimmin" for any of a number of reasons. They may be transgender or transsexual men, or they may be
genderqueers—not identifying as wimmin or men. There are a few intersex
conditions that might cause someone assigned male at birth to menstruate,
tied up in part with non-standard genitalia. And there are many intersex
people that menstruate and have complex organs. [Some of them are wimmin
are some are not.]

Non-menstruators who are wimmin come in lots of different kinds as well.
Some don't have vaginas, uteruses, fallopian tubes; some have some of those
organs but not the kind that would make them menstruate, like transsexual
wimmin and possibly some intersex folks. Some are young and have not
started to menstruate yet, and some are old and have gone through or are
going through menopause—the hormonal process that brings about an end to
menstruation, which usually happens between ages 40 and 55. Some people
don't menstruate because of illnesses, including eating disorders, or on
account of undergoing treatment or medication such as chemotherapy. Also
pregnant people usually don't menstruate, but sometimes they do bleed.
People who take certain types of chemical birth control, namely Depo-Provera
["the Shot"], may not menstruate or may menstruate very infrequently.

Irregular menstruation occurs most intensely in the first two years of menstruation and during menopause. Other common causes of irregularity are:
traveling; changes in sleep, diet, exercise; illness; stress; intense participation in
exercise/body movement; hormonal fluctuation from influences other than
pregnancy or birth control [such as hormone injections].[16]

The radical menstruation wing's careful thorough attention to degendering
menstruation stimulates a number of questions, among them, What is the effect
of making explicit the lack of universal correspondence between menstruation
and socially constructed womanhood? Put differently, What are the consequences
for political effectiveness when we make these exceptions explicit and adopt a
term that takes the "woman" out of menstruation? Is radical menstruation successful at drawing into the movement people who do not identify as women (but do
menstruate)? Are transpeople, intersexuals, and other gender-variant individuals
relieved to be acknowledged as menstruators?[17]

Throughout my research, I identified only two genderqueer or trans-identified
menstrual activists (EtShalom being one), although I met many self-identified
trans allies.[18] If transpeople were present at the actions I observed, they did not
make themselves known as such, so I began to ask menstrual activists to comment on the near invisibility of transpeople in the movement. Perhaps the movement wants to engage transpeople, but transpeople do not want the movement.
Believing the activist slogan "Nothing about us, without us," I set out to learn
about reactions to menstruation among trans-identified people.

Seeing Menstruation through Trans Eyes

For a woman who inhabits a biologically male body, the absence of menstruation may serve as a reminder of outsider status. And the presence of menstruation can be especially unwelcome for transmen. For example, for a man who inhabits a biologically female body, menstruation could serve as a marker of an identity that he has rejected. Holly Devor reports that menarche often initiates a major existential crisis for young transmen; in fact Devor found in her in-depth study of forty-five self-identified FtM transsexuals that "physiologically abnormal menses" were common among participants. Furthermore, "emotional resistance to menstruation was also a common theme among participants. Intensely negative sentiments were most common; fifty-one percent reported a high level of emotional discomfort about their menses. In some cases, these feelings were more connected to the social implications of physical maturation. In others, participants seemed to feel that the physical aspects of menstruation were both inappropriate to them and intrinsically defiling to them as human beings."[19]

In Henry Rubin's study, FtMs similarly "insist[ed] that their experiences [of menstruation] were uniquely awful, not at all ambivalent or tempered by positive emotions.[20] But other than noting the crisis of menarche and adolescent periods, none of the scholarly or popular literature on FtMs I located explores menstruation in any depth.

My research assistant Jessie Baird and I scoured trans-identified websites (including those devoted to trans health and various support and advocacy sites), open access discussion boards, and blogs to gather as much online information as possible about the transgendered body and menstruation before I approached transmen and requested interviews. We found very little. Menstruation seemed even more hidden in the transcommunity than in the general population.

The author of a website that explores how the medical community has shaped trans history explicitly encourages questions, except those that are "sexually curious." I wrote explaining my need for information related to the menstrual experiences of trans-identified people (and briefly explained my book project) and asked if she could direct me to an appropriate source. Several days later, I received the following reply:

> I've been holding off for days, trying to think of a response. When I offered to answer questions, it was about our political history, to help my community . . . and I specifically state that I would not answer sexually curious questions, which this certainly qualifies! First, I don't *ever* bring up subjects like this with the guys; . . . I mean . . . would I feel comfortable if one of them asked me a reciprocal question [and] . . . second, it reminded me, with very bad memories drug [sic] up, of an incident twenty-eight years ago when a transphobic neighbor called me, pretending to be a market researcher, asking the brand of tampons

I used. . . . HA HA HA . . . very funny . . . so it's rag on the pre-op male-to-female tranny day, HA HA!

My advice? Don't include transmen in your work . . . it would be demeaning to them. And frankly, also to Male-to-Female transwomen as well, . . . as the topic is defined as a "women's issue" . . . and pushing the transmen into that category hurts, but [sic] them and us, think about it for a moment. It would define FTM's as women and MTF's as not women. My request? Don't.[21]

This response stung and generated three interrelated responses. First, why did my contact respond so negatively? Upon reflection, the answer is obvious: There is little more disruptive to the social order than transgender existence, thus, transfolk must cultivate survivalist strategies to deflect unwanted attention and prurient interest. Further, given the strength of the menstrual taboo, any question of this nature may seem invasive and inappropriate, regardless of one's gender identity. (This may explain why my contact classified my menstruation-related question as "sexually curious.") Thus, what might initially come across as defensiveness is no doubt legitimate self-protection. Second, the conclusion that menstruation defines FtMs as women and MtFs as men was a poignant reflection of the socially determined meaning of menstruation. And third, my contact's request that I not pursue my research caused me to pause. Together with Jessie, I struggled with this for quite some time. Should I, in good faith as a trans ally, drop this search for information? If a transperson, in particular an expert in transgender history and someone committed to increasing trans visibility and support, registered such a strong negative reaction to my query, perhaps I should take heed.

Ultimately, I decided not to conduct in-depth interviews with trans-identified people, given my own gender identity, lack of contacts in transcommunities, and the considerations just outlined; I feared that my requests for interviews would come across as intrusive, even exploitative. However, I remained committed to capturing even an extremely partial sense of the interface between menstruation and the trans experience, so that I could more knowledgably explore the dimension of transinclusion in subsequent interviews with radical menstruation activists.

To this end, Jessie and I posted what we hoped were sensitively worded queries on a number of open-access trans-supportive message boards. We reasoned that since posters maintained anonymity on the boards and could ignore any post (many more bizarre than ours), responding to our queries was a relatively low-impact, low-risk task. I realized that any information we gathered could not be construed as representative, nor could the authenticity of the postings be verified, but I hoped to gain insight into how some trans-identified people reckon with the topic of menstruation. It was a beginning.

The tone of the responses to menstruation we received ranged from detached disinterest to outright hostility. While the questions offended some people, others expressed interest in this topic and were willing to share their stories.

On one message board, the first respondent, a self-identified biological woman, volunteered how awful it is to menstruate: "I am a GG [genetic girl] and let me tell you . . . it sucks!!" An MtF wrote back: "But see? You have something to talk about with regards to that and I can only try to imagine what it's like." Expressing a similar sentiment, a postoperative MtF wrote: "I will never know what it feels like to menstruate or to carry a child. When I do think of these things I feel saddened and cheated. Genetic women tell me how lucky I am not to get a period. But I don't feel lucky . . . I will never get to know what every other woman does." Wrestling with the weight of menstruation in shaping her identity, she continued: "Does getting a period or having a baby [or lack thereof] make any of us more or less women? There are a lot of genetic females who no longer get their period, and this does not in the least bit make them any less of a woman. But still . . ." In response, another poster stated that "it's not the fact that we need to feel the effects of Menses—but we need to feel akin to other women," and another that "not being able to bear children is one of the worst consequences of having been born this way," and "it's a hard and cruel topic." On a different note, a respondent offered that some MtFs vary their doses of estrogen during the month to simulate the menstrual cycle. Finally, a poster suggested that information of this kind "should be in a seminar somewhere for TS [transsexuals]," and that "it sure isn't being talked about in the support groups up here in ND [North Dakota]."

These responses, rich with emotion, demonstrate the strength of the link between the embodied experience of menstruation and identity. Notably, all responses were posted by either biological or transsexual women. Not one self-identified transman offered a view or an experience. Are transmen, including those who have menstruated and continue to do so, silent on this issue? Is discussing it too painful, too fraught? If so, are menstrual activists reaching out to a disinterested population, or worse, by articulating that some transmen might menstruate, calling attention to the very embodied limits of the female-to-male transition? With these questions in mind, I began asking activists in the field to respond to the information we had gathered.

RESPONSES OF RADICAL MENSTRUATION ACTIVISTS

During a group interview with nine student menstrual activists at Macalester College in St. Paul, Minnesota, I described the kind of resistance Jessie and I met when we broached the topic of menstruation online and asked: "What, from your perspective, is the point of working to include transfolks in the menstrual activism movement?" One of the activists, a young woman named Abby Woodworth majoring in women's and gender studies, reframed the issue, specifying trans agency: "It's still really important to be giving groups the opportunity to decide if they want *you* to become part of *their* movement." Another activist, Sarah

Claasen, agreed and shared a recent realization: "I am recognizing that as a [trans] ally, the [trans] movement is not made for me," thus suggesting that as a nontrans menstrual activist, it is her responsibility to respect the needs and priorities of transpeople, even if an issue dear to her—menstruation—is not among those priorities. The issue is not whether transpeople want to be a part of the menstrual activist movement, but whether the members of the trans movement want to include menstrual issues. Another student, Maggie Kinkead, who had earlier disclosed that, although a healthy biological woman, she does not menstruate, echoed this same sentiment by telling transpeople: "We are not forcing Tampaction [the SEAC campaign] on you, but here we are." Activist Jo Williams chimed in that "because trans is so much about passing, it is important to keep the focus on 'nobody gets to tell you how to be a man or a woman.'"[22] And this makes the key point: Using the language "menstruator" is not only about trans outreach, but also about using gender-neutral language to queer the gender binary, as Williams went on to note: "We talk about menstruators, not women, because we are doing more than creating space for more people, but we are queering gender too."

Emerging in the context of feminism's third wave, this is gender theory in practice, a point echoed in a group interview with Fort Collins, Colorado, student and community-based activists. Michelle, a local activist and graduate of Colorado State University who studied feminist philosophy, explained that using the language "menstruator" rather than "woman" presents an opportunity to educate others about the fluidity of gender. Every time the word "menstruator" is uttered, she told me, it disrupts our normative conceptions of bodies, which calls into question the biological definitions at the root of gender in Western culture. For her, this linguistic choice is an important part of "doing gender education," which fundamentally seeks to undo gender as we know it.

TROUBLING GENDER THROUGH RADICAL MENSTRUATION

Making linguistic choices such as shifting from "women" to "menstruators" signals the inclusion fundamental to third-wave feminism. Borrowing from Pandora Leong, contributor to *Colonize This: Young Women of Color on Today's Feminism*, who advocates "making room for everyone under the feminist tent," we need a tent that covers as many genders as there are people: transgender, androgyne, intergender, bigender, bio, third gender, neuter/neutrois/agender, genderqueer, and gender fluid, and more, say third-wavers.[23] The many linkages between third-wave feminism and transgender theorizing and activism demonstrate that the grounds for inclusion in gender theorizing are much broader than originally conceived. However, some feminists are not ready to redraw the lines. Some in the transcommunity, like trans historian Susan Stryker, align with third-wave feminism as a reaction against the transphobia associated with at least some corners of second-wave feminism, such as Janice Raymond's notoriously extreme position against transsexuality. This anti-trans sentiment, claims Stryker, is "an unfortunate consequence of the second-wave feminist turn to an untheorised female body as the ultimate ground for feminist practice." The third wave, however, situated in the postmodern context that reenvisions relationships between sex, the body, and gender, is more equipped to carry trans issues forward. Stryker writes, in terms both grandiose and (by her own admission) esoteric: "Within the feminist third-wave . . . transgender phenomena have come to constitute important evidence in recent arguments about essentialism and social constructionism, performativity and citationality, hybridity and fluidity, anti-foundational ontologies and non-referential epistemologies, the proliferation of perversities, the collapse of difference, the triumph of technology, the advent of posthumanism and the end of the world as we know it." As Stryker notes, transgender theorizing is not only significant because it prescribes transgender liberation but also because it enriches and complicates extant debates across many fields of inquiry.[24]

But using gender-neutral language to contest the dominant cultural narrative of menstruation is complicated, perhaps contradictory, work. Does this intimidate the radical menstruation activists? No. Since they take their cue from third-wave feminism, which works with rather than against contradictions, the messiness of degendering menstruation is an invitation to, not a disincentive for, engagement. Perhaps the word most often used to characterize third-wave feminism is "contradiction," as I suggest in chapter 1. Indeed, third-wavers reckon with unwieldy incongruities as essential to building an authentically diverse movement, at both conceptual and practical levels. The radical menstruation activists delight in the complex implications that queering menstrual talk produces. On the one hand, they attack FemCare exploitation of women's bodies for profit. On the other, they refuse to frame menstruation as a women-only issue, which they argue just reifies the oppressive gender binary at the root of social injustice for women *and* men. Can they have it both ways? Can they afford not to?

In the world of contemporary feminism, the term "troubling gender"—most readily (though certainly not exclusively) associated with feminist/queer theorist Judith Butler—is nearly a household phrase. In Butler's pathbreaking 1990 book *Gender Trouble: Feminism and the Subversion of Identity*, she describes gender categories as constructed and reconstructed through historically and culturally embedded discourses and thus always unstable. She explains in a later book what motivated her to write *Gender Trouble*: "My effort was to combat forms of essentialism which claimed that gender is a truth that is somehow there, interior to the body, as a core or as an internal essence, something that we cannot deny, something which, natural or not, is treated as a given."[25]

When Butler theorizes that sex itself is also socially constructed as little more than a discursive artifact, she separates herself from the pack of feminist sociologists who concur on the well-established social construction of gender such as Judith Lorber, Barbara Risman, Barrie Thorne, Candace West, and Don Zimmerman. According to Butler: "There is no recourse to a body that has already been interpreted by cultural meanings, hence sex could not qualify as a prediscursive anatomical facticity."[26] For Butler, bodies cannot be unproblematically defined by certain capacities, for example, pregnancy: "Why is it pregnancy by which [woman's] body gets defined? One might say it's because somebody is of a given sex that they go to the gynecologist to get an examination that establishes the possibility of pregnancy or one might say that going to the gynecologist is the very production of 'sex,' but it is still the question of pregnancy that is centering the whole institutional practice here."[27] For Butler, questions of biological differences are not fundamentally questions about the materiality of the body but questions that discursively reinforce the norm, only asserting the salience of the social institution of reproduction. That is, when pregnancy is held up as proof of sexual difference, it proves only the strength of cultural norms, not the intractability of difference. Menstruation similarly proves how biological capacities are used in the service of creating and reinforcing the bifurcated gender paradigm, which, according to Butler, is foundational to heteronormativity.[28]

Judith Butler's theorizing contrasts with that of sexual difference theorists such as Rosi Braidotti, who reject the concept of gender instability as a politically disastrous erasure of the category "woman." For them, various acts that affirm femininity are most effective at mobilizing women as political agents. This strain of the theory pursues the development of female subjectivity through the annunciation of sexual differences, seen through a feminist lens as positive and agentic, as Braidotti explains in *Nomadic Subjects: Embodiment and Sexual Difference in Feminist Theory*: "I have opted for the extreme affirmation of a sexed identity as a way of reversing the attribution of difference in a hierarchical mode. This extreme affirmation of sexual difference may lead to repetition, but the crucial factor here is that it empowers women to act."[29]

Judith Butler's theorizing of gender, however, has captured the third-wave feminist imaginary, catapulting her to cultlike status among students of feminist theory who reject positions like those of Braidotti and other sexual differences theorists. Reading Butler has become a rite of passage for students of feminist theory. Even students who take only one or a few women's or gender studies classes most likely encounter her ideas, if indirectly. Of the radical menstruation activists I interviewed, 72 percent took at least one women's or gender studies course, an experience made obvious in the ways their understandings of the volatile nature of gender shaped their menstrual activism (see chapter 5). Radical menstruation activists like EtShalom, Fawn P., and Marie Abbondanza, and numerous campus activists affiliated with SEAC's Tampaction campaign, "live Butler" by applying her ideas to their activism. They simultaneously do public health and subvert the gender order.

WHITHER IDENTITY POLITICS?

I must make clear that "living Butler" as a way of "doing feminism" is limited (in the arena of menstrual activism) to those affiliated with the radical menstruation wing of the movement.[30] The feminist-spiritualists do not trouble gender. Like sexual difference theorists, the destabilization of subjective identity poses problems for them. Their activism rests on the conceptualization of women's interests, issues, and concerns that cannot be easily articulated, let alone defended, if the central subject is eroded, removing the basis for political action—a circumstance that would, as J. Ransom puts it, "disappear the hook on which to hang our feminism."[31]

The tension between feminist-spiritualists' and radical menstruation activists' conceptualizations regarding the category "woman" reflects a larger tension that sits at the center of Western feminist theorizing, as I have stated. For at least twenty years, scholars have found this tension a fruitful theme.[32] The debate boils down to two questions: First, does effective political action depend on a strategic essentialism? Second, if not, what is the future of identity-based movements like feminism? Rachel Alsop, Annette Fitzsimons, and Kathleen Lennon effectively summarize the terms of the debate: "The current anti-essentialist mood within gender theory, fuelled by the recognition of differences between women as well as the insights of deconstructionism and queer analysis, challenges the very foundations of identity-based political movements, such as the feminist women's movement, and therefore raises crucial questions about political agency and intervention."[33]

Sociologist Josh Gamson works through the good, the bad, and the ugly of identity politics by examining the contentious debate over the loaded word "queer" in the LGBTQ movement: Shall we reclaim it or bury it? He concludes that the logics of both perspectives are "true, and neither is fully tenable." In his view: "*Secure boundaries and stabilized identities are necessary, not in the general, but in the specific*—a point which current social movement theory largely misses; . . . the American political environment makes stable collective identities both necessary and damaging."[34]

While Gamson's argument is compelling, its abstractness prevents one from fully grasping how the difference between the strategic essentialists and the gender troublemakers translates into practice. This is precisely why I find the tension between the two wings of the movement especially useful. The contrast between the feminist-spiritualists and the radical menstruation activists—in terms of their divergent ways of framing the relationships among gender, the body, and menstruation—produce very different plans of action. The feminist-spiritualists draw strength from their identities as women, and they seek to recuperate a power attached to essential embodiment destroyed by patriarchy.

The radical menstruation activists sever the naturalized link between embodiment and gender—not only because doing so is consistent with their aspiration to be fully inclusive, but also because it supports the third-wave agenda of blurring boundaries, defying categorization, and embracing contradiction more generally. Putting gender theory to the test, they deconstruct the gender binary at the level of the body without relinquishing political agency.

But there remains between the two wings of the menstrual activist movement a trench that reflects in microcosm a chasm within feminism. Can this space be bridged? Is it possible to simultaneously acknowledge real social, political, and cultural forces that continue to shape the menstrual experience in destructive and oppressive ways without falling into the treacherous essentialist trap that locates identity in the biological body?

The work of Diana Fuss is helpful in imagining beyond the metabinary of sexual difference or gender theory. She asserts in her influential book *Essentially Speaking: Feminism, Nature, and Difference* that feminist action is neither the denial nor the affirmation of embodied differences, but rather the working knowledge that changes in social, economic, political, and historical contexts produce them. That is, a feminist future depends not on erasing or celebrating sexed differences but on producing a collective consciousness that theorizes and acts on social processes and their implications. Butler herself suggests that proving the substance of sexual difference is a difficult task, so we are well advised to "make no decision what sexual difference is but leave that question open, troubling, unresolved, propitious."[35]

But what do we do about language? Theorists have the luxury of patience, but activists must make strategic decisions in the moment. They have zines to write, workshops to advertise, and roadshows to plan. While I think there is room in the movement for both approaches, I prefer the radical menstruation approach of referring to "menstruators" while slowly nudging the feminist-spiritualists to expand the category "woman" until it breaks. In the meantime, perhaps the menstrual activism movement, unified by the shared goal of challenging the dominant cultural narrative of menstruation—and by extension, of feminism generally—can grow stronger and more powerful through, not in spite of, its intramovement ideological and tactical differences.

I suspect the Bloodsisters would agree. They tuned into the diversity of approaches to menstrual activism long before I began my research, as this passage from a zine suggests:

We are feminist terrorists
We are quiet moss bleeders
We are riot grrrl boy catchers
We are goddess thumpers
We are bloody Punk rockers
We are moon worshippers
We are terrible singers
We are dirty girl power.[36]

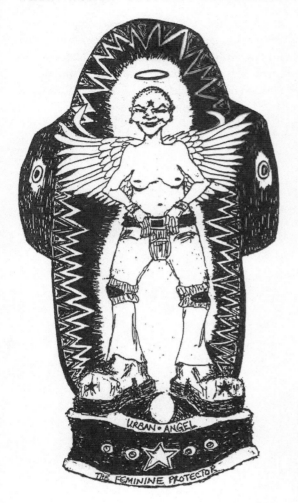

Figure 11. adee and Danielle, "Urban Angel: The Feminine Protector," 1996. Courtesy of adee (conception) and Danielle (execution) (The Bloodsisters Project).

With these words, they imply that the menstrual activism movement must make room for a diverse range of perspectives and expressions, from "moon worshippers" to "bloody punk rockers." The gender-bending character "Urban Angel: The Feminine Protector," also a Bloodsisters "reproduction" (many of their visual materials are thus labeled), is a playful representation of the blending of goddess and punk, invoking Mexican iconography of the Virgin of Guadalupe.[37] Framed by a cloth menstrual pad (with snaps) and firmly planted atop a pedestal, she is "here to protect" (an obvious play on "sanitary protection"). Since 1994, "Urban Angel," active, defiant, and confrontational, revels in rich contradictions: bad-ass attitude encircled with a dainty halo, delicate wings paired with oversized combat boots, bald, butch, and breasted. Radical menstruation activists are skilled at presenting us with the unexpected. Their tactics are leading the menstrual activism movement to the cutting edge, where we can more clearly see the relationship of sex to gender and can challenge the binaries behind *all* the -isms. Furthermore and even more crucially, these activists show us how third-wave feminism, indebted to a rich tradition in feminist theory, is smashing categories along the way to social justice.

Conclusion

A year after meeting the Bloodsisters and beginning my research into menstrual activism, I have returned to the this increasingly controversial feminist event. Here, the womyn-born-womyn policy that excludes transwomen is all the buzz, and perhaps nothing more clearly demonstrates that feminism as we know it is in a state of crisis. The policy articulates the palpable tension between those who wish to preserve womanhood as a core category of feminism and those who wish to explode not only that category, but also the gender binary on which it rests. Will this dilemma ultimately destroy the movement or strengthen it? I take the latter position. In fact, the crisis energizes and reassures me. I have the menstrual activists to thank for that. Since getting to know the people and the ideas associated with this little known but nonetheless potent movement, I have uncharacteristically become an optimist.

This perspective crystallizes on Wednesday evening during my first experience in a mosh pit, the site of the energetic, pushing-shoving-jumping style of dancing typical of punk and heavy metal shows. Though I am anxious, I am surrounded by women mostly in their twenties who are clearly big fans of the band onstage. I am a fortunate neophyte, for by all accounts, this is a very friendly pit comparatively speaking. Women even help you up when you fall down.

The band onstage is the Butchies, a punk rock trio comprised of self-described butch dykes Kaia Wilson, Melissa York, and Alison Metlew. I am immediately drawn into their politicized high energy and unabashedly queer music. While the Butchies are relatively new to me, their record label—Mr. Lady Records—is not. Band member Kaia Wilson and her girlfriend, Tammy Rae Carland, founded the independent feminist lesbian company in 1996 as a key recording outlet for "queercore" bands.

With their next number, I experience a flash of recognition. The song is a hyper, electric-guitar-styled cover of "Shooting Star"—the Cris Williamson classic I know well from the early heady days of women's music. Williamson recorded "Shooting Star" in 1975 on her much-celebrated first album, *Changer and the Changed*, one of Olivia Records' first releases. The founders of Olivia, the first recording label for explicitly lesbian musical talent, were pioneers; their label was indie before indie was hip and women's music was an established genre. Knowing the rich history this music represents, I am impressed and delighted that the Butchies chose to cover this tune. It points—quite literally— to the interplay of continuity and change expressed in contemporary feminism, and this, I believe, promises a vibrant future for the movement.

Close inspection of the people, ideas, and actions at menstrual activism's core has taught me a lot about feminism today. Through the menstrual activists, I was able not only to relate what's exciting and different about contemporary expressions of feminism, but also to reveal an interesting story of continuity. Today's feminism on the ground embodies a set of ideological departures that require practical innovation, such as the way radical menstruation activists queer gender by referring to "menstruators," not "women." At the same time, the movement's third wave is deeply indebted to its past, especially at the tactical level. Zines, street theatre, workshopping, and DIY health care all have precedents in the second wave. Put simply, the content may be shifting, but the forms are largely the same. This wasn't obvious to me at first.

Attracted by the sassy "Pussy Power" t-shirts paired with miniskirts and bright lipstick, by stylized zines and angry anticorporate posters scrawled in red paint, I assumed that menstrual activism was a third-wave brainchild—funky, fresh, edgy, and new. But I discovered, as I dug beneath the aesthetic, that the movement has a history reaching back into the early 1970s and that radical menstruation—its most recent manifestation—is merely one among several feminist activist expressions engaging menstruation. There were the early cultural feminists like renegade filmmaker Emily Culpepper and pioneering artist Judy Chicago, who were soon joined by feminist health activists, environmentalists, and consumer rights advocates set on fire by the underregulated FemCare industry. And, in the mid-1970s, feminist-spiritualist pioneers like Tamara Slayton and Jeannine Parvati began shaking up the thinking about the place of menstruation in women's lives and established a tradition that endures—if only marginally—today.

But the radical menstruation activists I met were largely ignorant of the roots of their movement. When I share this news with fellow feminist scholars and writers, they typically shake their heads. "See? I told you we were in trouble!" They worry that this impoverished historical understanding bodes poorly for feminism. Movement strength depends on preserving its own institutional memory, doesn't it? Second-wave feminists knew this when they intentionally self-identified as second-wave because they wished to explicitly articulate a connection to their past, as Amber Kinser suggests: "The second-wave attention to women's rights, and more importantly, to women's liberation, emerged seemingly out of nowhere and needed to re-establish itself as neither particularly new nor fleeting. The labeling that linked the two periods of feminist movement was a rhetorical strategy that helped give clout to '60s women's activism and positioned it as a further evolution of the earlier and larger movement."[1]

The deployment of the wave metaphor in the label "third-wave feminism" implies continuity with an already established movement. But given the amount of distance third-wavers put between themselves and their second-wave mothers, there's something different going on here. Third-wave feminists self-consciously highlight their differences from the second wave. They, as I have said, advance an us/them construction that worries some second-wavers, who see such a differentiation as based on a profound ignorance of the past.

The second-wave claim that the third wave has a distorted view of its immediate predecessors finds support in my analysis of contemporary menstrual activism, especially among the radical menstruation activists (the Bloodsisters, acutely aware of the fertile soil that sprouted their particular late twentieth-century contributions, are an exception). Although this finding does not alarm me, it frustrates me, and it raises questions. Is the third-wave's ahistoricity a failure of the women's movement to keep its history alive? Or is this historical blindness simply the consequence of the short attention span of youth and the deep—and developmentally appropriate—need for independence and self-definition? My data do not answer these questions, but I hope feminist historians will pursue this line of inquiry.

For me, the more urgent question it this: Does third-wave resistance to the second wave portend the death of feminism? While salivating social conservatives, body bag at the ready, are keen to pronounce feminism dead, I find in the third wave's break with the past—in contrast to the second wave's embrace of its feminist history—a signal of the movement's vitality. Unlike feminists who came of age in the 1960s, third-wavers are not emerging out of nowhere (even if "nowhere" is an exaggeration, as scholars of the in-between years, namely Verta Taylor and Leila Rupp, demonstrate).[2] Amy Richards and Jennifer Baumgardner famously wrote that for today's youth, "feminism is like fluoride. We scarcely notice we have it— it's simply in the water."[3] We are surrounded by evidence of the tremendous successes of the second wave; the problem isn't that feminism is nowhere, but that it is everywhere. This is a good problem to have. Call off the autopsy.

What Now?

In a question-and-answer period following a lecture I gave not long ago, a highly esteemed feminist sociologist queried regarding the "queering gender" project of third-wave feminists: "I am terrified. Where are we going?" Where *are* we going?" As she spoke, her voice quivered. I understand her anxiety. How do we get there when we are not in agreement about where "there" is? Are we ready to undo gender when gender discrimination is still practiced everywhere, everyday? How do we acknowledge and name even relatively minor biological differences without losing sight of the much bigger differences we socially construct? Are our categories an unwieldy necessity, or is progress elusive if we do not undo gender? Many of us are asking such questions.

Critical race scholars, for example, are similarly struggling over what do about the concept "race." In "Buried Alive: The Concept of Race in Science," sociologist Troy Duster argues that calls to discard the concept are premature. Although race as a construct may be little more than a social convention (and, says Duster, "the diabolical Siamese twin of racism"), we can not pronounce it dead—not yet. Instead, he advocates a trenchant interrogation of the complex relationship between the social and the biological: "It is a mistake to discard race just because racial categories do not map exactly onto biological processes. But it is also a mistake to uncritically accept old racial classifications."[4] If race is an imperfect yet still necessary category, can we say the same for gender in the context of feminist activism? This question is much easier to entertain in the abstract, and that is precisely why I choose to pose it in the context of a social movement centered on the material body.

Through menstrual activism, the problems become very real. In contemporary menstrual activism, there are two models of negotiating gender. The ideology of the first centers on the reclamation of womanhood *as* a central category. Gendering menstruation, in the tradition of the feminist-spiritualists, helps us see the sexism that drives menstrual discourse and practice, although their take on gender, as I've shown, is raced and classed in ways that exclude. The ideology the second—degendering menstruation, radical menstruation–style—bursts the boundaries of the movement (and feminism more generally) at the same time it questions the gender binary. This act tears at the fabric from which we construct the punishing straitjackets of hegemonic masculinity and femininity. But like feminist-spiritualists, radical menstruation activists have not yet built a movement that attracts a rich diversity of participants. Contesting categories is unsettling, and at times the debates seem endless, unresolvable. I realized early in my research that even though I talked the talk of shifting boundaries and unstable constructs, I was invested in categorization; indeed, my research was fundamentally a quest for *more* categories, including the category "menstrual activist" that I later learned was capturing an overwhelmingly white and middle-class population.[5] I remember my unease in an early interview with Lily, a radical menstruation activist. When I asked her my open-ended lead question, "How would you describe yourself?" she replied: "How do I identity myself? I don't feel like answering this one—knock me out with the first punch! It's too easy of an out to say that I don't like defining myself or putting people in boxes because as we all know, that's idealistic and not useful anyway. But as a caveat, I'm not stuck on any way of defining myself these days."[6] For Lily, my question asked her to set limits. And she was right. I *was* searching for a way to peg her: feminist? environmentalist? rebel? earth mother? Her refusal to play along with my reductive game challenged me at first. Lily, like many others I met, refused to work within categories. Instead, she was, to paraphrase another menstrual activist, "doing the feminist business of crossing lines."

Lily and others set me on a path of discovery, and with time, I came to feel less frustrated and more energized. I began to see third-wave feminism vis-à-vis menstrual activism as a model of how not only to challenge the status quo that oppresses, but also to push back against the categories at the foundation of injustice. Although menstrual activism has its weaknesses—its whiteness (at least on the surface), its privilege, its under-the-radar status—and some will rightly challenge some of its tactics, it does illustrate what "doing feminism" looks like when fundamental categories are troubled. Further, it demonstrates evidence of feminism's dynamic energy. When feminism is bold enough, even confident enough, to engage in this kind of self-reflection and revision, we all benefit. The challenge is to make feminism relevant, to make it speak up where it has been silent. This is the work of menstrual activism. And we need menstrual activism now more than ever.

Here's an example of what's at stake: A recent commercial for Barr Pharmaceuticals' Seasonique (an oral contraceptive that limits menstrual periods to four per year) opens with two women greeting one another, one on either side of a split screen. "Hey, Logical!" says woman #1. "Hey, Emotional!" cheerfully replies woman #2. Quickly, it becomes obvious that Logical and Emotional are aspects of the same woman, one skeptical and serious, the other, carefree and fun. So that the viewer doesn't miss the contrast, Logical wears brown pants, a white blouse, and an argyle vest. Her long straight hair is neatly combed and partly pulled back. Emotional wears a jewel-toned blouse with a ruffle at its hem, jeans, and a long necklace. Her hair is wavy and a bit windswept. The commercial proceeds with Emotional trying to convince Logical of the merits of "birth control with fewer periods." As a voiceover runs through a dizzying series of product disclaimers, Logical thoughtfully studies the Seasonique webpage on her laptop while Emotional spins playfully in a chair, tries to engage Logical in a game of ball, and dances in a flouncy dress. In the end, Logical literally crosses over to Emotional's side of the screen and *becomes* Emotional. The woman's choice is obvious: "birth control with fewer periods." In this commercial, Logical represents the so-called thinking woman who has her doubts about the logic of suppressing menstruation, but Emotional prevails. It is not hard to imagine Emotional's unspoken argument: "Come on! Why not? Don't be so old-fashioned! You know you want to get rid of your period! Periods hold us back! Periods aren't fun! You're a liberated woman—act like one!"[7]

I find this commercial distressing not only because it artificially splits the emotional from the logical and forces a choice between two interdependent aspects of the human psyche, but also because it illustrates so transparently what makers of pills that suppress menstruation know so well. Seasonique and other cycle-stopping contraceptives are appealing because they tap into women's deep *emotional* reactions to menstruation. The FemCare industry, of course, has exploited the menstrual taboo and a lack of information surrounding menstruation for decades. Now, the pharmaceutical industry is on board, too. Cleverly, however, Seasonique's ad doesn't explicitly invoke the taboo but subtly reduces the issue of menstrual suppression to a conflict between head and heart. As the Society for Menstrual Cycle Research points out, the long-term safety of cycle-stopping contraception is still unknown. It might be safe, but it might not; it is too soon to tell. Provisional industry-sponsored research cannot credibly assure consumers of the long-term safety of what is nothing more, in most instances, than a lifestyle drug. But do most women considering menstrual suppression know about the inadequacy of the available data? I doubt it.

What women do know is this: Menstruation is a hassle, and technology gives women freedom. The newest continuous-use contraceptive was named Lybrel to invoke "liberty," say product makers.[8] Cunning. But how free is choice making in the dark? How can we genuinely choose anything at all if we aren't clear on the nature of the options before us? Somebody needs to turn on the lights to reveal the whole story. And when those of us who question menstrual suppression do finally flip the switch, we find ourselves with some strange bedfellows.

On the heels of FDA approval of Lybrel, a cartoon by Ann Telnaes appeared in the Internet-based feminist newsmagazine *Women's eNews*. A woman reads a newspaper whose headline reads: "FDA approves birth control pill that blocks menstruation." A pair of protestors—a man and a woman, both conservatively dressed—stoically stand nearby holding a sign: "Life Begins at Menstruation." The woman reading the newspaper says, without looking up, "Give it a rest." This sly joke jabs at the antiabortion discursive strategy of definitional creep. A woman's body is not her own; goes the polemic; it is a vessel that contains new life. Extend this reasoning and even the uterine lining is sacred and must be preserved. Menstrual suppression, in this fictional (I hope) view, is murder. But the woman reading the newspaper will have none of it. Enough already, she says. Back off! It's just a period! And, from that perspective, the comic is funny. From a menstrual activist standpoint, however, the implications are not too humorous.

While I am quite certain that no critic of menstrual suppression regards cycle-stopping contraception as an appropriate new battlefield in the abortion war, there are many who would agree that the menstrual cycle should be defended, or at least not so easily dismissed. Many menstrual activists are troubled that Big Pharma encourages increasing numbers of women to breezily reject a fundamental biological process, rendering it passé for today's "liberated" woman—obviously

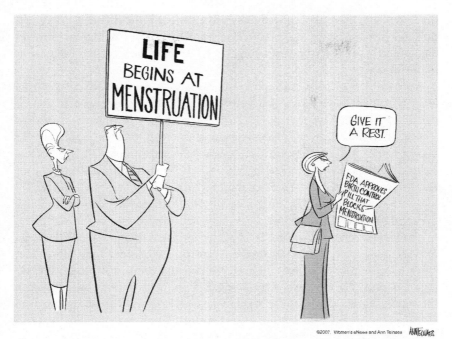

Figure 12. Ann Telnaes, "Life Begins at Menstruation," 2007. Used with the permission of Ann Telnaes and Women's eNews in conjunction with the Cartoonist Group. All rights reserved.

a second-wave construct (think women's "lib") that still has resonance even in today's third wave. But hold on a minute, say the menstrual activists; respecting the physiological, emotional, and practical dimensions of the menstrual cycle is very good feminist practice that prioritizes caring for our bodies over ceding to social taboos. Nevertheless, we must tread this path carefully. Responsible menstrual activism requires advancing an alternative view of menstruation without unwittingly falling into the potholes of essentialist romanticism or biological determinism. We cannot allow menstrual activist discourse to be exploited to perpetuate business (*yes, business*) as usual.

Women, as agents of their lives, have a right to control all aspects of their bodies, especially their reproduction. For me, it boils down to the classic pro-choice slogan, "My Body, My Choice," with a twist. It might be clunky and ill suited to clever chants and cheers, but might the slogan more usefully expand to say, "My Right to Information, My Body, My Choice"? Without comprehensive data from thorough, high-quality, independent longitudinal research, menstrual suppression for nonmedical indications is risky. Menstrual activists of all stripes concede that menstruation poses a problem (physiological and beyond) for many, even most, menstruators, but they emphasize the role our cultural attitudes play in shaping the experience of menstruation. The biggest problem is not menstruation, per se, they say, but an enduring tradition that pathologizes women's bodies and regards *all* bodies as objects in constant need of (commodified) improvement.

Since the introduction of commercial FemCare, the industry has co-opted the feminist rhetoric of freedom. Today, pharmaceutical companies peddling menstrual suppression have joined in. The noise generated by industry-sponsored clinical trials and a seemingly endless string of prosuppression articles in the mainstream press reduces critics of cycle-stopping contraception to puritans, fundamentalists, and chauvinists.[9] This talk effectively drowns out calls to proceed with caution or for the application of what the public health advocates call the precautionary principle, which places the burden of proof on those who risk the public health."[10] Is the situation as untenable as it seems?

The way out of this impasse is to step back and ask some questions. What does it mean to be liberated? What does it mean to be an agent of one's own life? Various answers to these questions have formed a cornerstone of feminist thinking and doing since the dawn of the women's movement. The first-wave focus on suffrage and property rights, the second-wave focus on violence against women and on sexual politics, and the third-wave focus on the everyday and the instability of categories—all are grounded in the trenchant feminist belief that each woman (increasingly, each *person*) can and should determine who she (or he) is and how she (or he) shall live. That is, to be truly free, one must possess the power to make choices in one's own best interest. This is agency. This is liberation.

But how can someone truly decide what is best without all the information one needs to fully weigh the pros and cons? What kind of freedom is that? How free are we if we express this so-called liberation through denying the self in response to social pressures on the run from a deeply entrenched taboo? The *authentic* choice for menstrual suppression, then, is a choice based on solid, reliable, objective information. It is not a mad dash away from a bodily process shrouded in misunderstanding and silence.

This kind of questioning is critical if—as feminists and as people who work for progressive social transformation—we are to stay honest with ourselves and each other. A close look at menstrual activism over time reveals a good model of how to do this. Through a lens on the menstrual activists, especially the radical menstruation wing, the imperative to probe beneath the surface comes into focus. The menstrual activists show us that when we interrogate the relationships between the material body and identity, the cultural and the biological, and the social and the individual—and even when we question the very categories upon which the movement itself rests—we are better equipped to make profound change. Listen to the menstrual activists. They are living this transformation-in-progress.

Sharon Powell, "the Coochie Lady," is a menstrual activist who herself defies categorization. She is an African American women's health educator, poet, and performer who fits tidily in neither the feminist-spiritualist nor the radical menstruation wing of the movement. For that reason, I find her words especially compelling. During our interview, her response to my concluding interview question, "Where is menstrual activism headed?" resonated well beyond the movement to transform menstrual culture and practice. Because it speaks to the future of feminism as dependent on the thoughtful and thorough questioning of, as she puts, "what we think we know," the last word is hers: "As long as we continue to be socialized in a way that creates an environment where menstrual bleeding is yucky, a bother, and something that interferes unnecessarily with my good time, then we are in trouble. I am hopeful, however, that as we truly share information and skills, and encourage people to interrogate what we think we know, this will change. Not just for menstrual cycle work, but for everything."[11]

Appendix A. Methods

ACCESSING THE FIELD AND DATA COLLECTION

ACCESSING THE FIELD AND DATA COLLECTION

Getting to know the menstrual activists, past and present, demanded multiple methods. Since no one had conducted an in-depth study devoted exclusively to menstrual activism, I was aware that a combination of qualitative approaches would be necessary to fully represent and interpret this understudied social movement. Thus this work is at once a textual analysis of movement materials, a sociologically informed ethnography, and a historical investigation that mines archival sources.

In the fall of 2002 I began collecting menstrual activist materials, including menstrually themed zines, and exploring e-zines and websites (blogs were just beginning to emerge). Some of the earlier zines were produced in the mid to late 1990s; others were quite recent. Because of their ephemeral nature, I was not always able to secure every zine I had read about in other zines, found in catalogues of zine distribution services (called "distros"), or heard described by activists themselves. Nonetheless, I collected twenty-five zines and ten e-zines or websites (the difference between the two is not always clear) with menstrual heath and politics at their center. Using this material, I performed a textual analysis that enabled me to identify themes threaded through contemporary movement discourse. The textual analysis also helped me locate the movement organizations that feed menstrual activism—women's health collectives, student environmental groups, artists' collectives, punk and anarchist groups, and feminist spirituality communities.

I invited the creators of the zines, e-zines, and websites I was able to contact for in-depth interviews and interviewed ten of them—my first set of interviews, which helped me hone the questions that drove the next phase of my research project: participant observation.

I knew that I, a white, (at the time) forty-two-year-old college professor and married suburban mother of two, would not immediately fit in with hip punk, anarchist, urban young women. I knew our clothes, our hair, our means of making a living, and our musical tastes, at the very least, would differ dramatically (even if many of our social analyses converged). I doubted if I could skillfully minimize those differences and capitalize on our commonalities.

My first encounter was with a small group of Boston-based young punk women who founded a short-lived punk rock feminist collective, Moshtrogen. I was interested in this group because they produced a zine that included substantial menstrual health and politics content and they gave local workshops on radical menstruation. I gained access to them through a student of mine, an occasional member of the group, whom I met, my heart beating a mile a minute, at the subway station near the host's house (a large house shared by several twenty-somethings, both men and women). As we entered the rather rough-and-tumble house with a gaggle of bikes nearly blocking the front door, I felt out of place. We sat down in the living room (filled with mismatched secondhand furniture, a painted bed sheet hanging on the wall); my unease grew. As the room began to fill with the collective's members and in spite of a series of warm greetings, I was aware that my jeans and t-shirt contrasted with the layered and ripped shirts and hoodies, skirts over patched pants, thick boots, creative accessories—many borrowed from little girl culture—and even more creative hairstyles adorning the young women facing me. It was clear that I would have to find a way to connect with my informants without misrepresenting who I was. There was no hiding my age (or my privilege), but I could make it clear that my interest in the work of menstrual activism was genuine and, at the data collection phase at least, I was not in the business of making judgments. The meeting went well (entirely to the credit of my hosts); the young women were forthcoming about their work and excited about my research. They invited me to an upcoming event and promised to add me to their e-mail discussion list. I realized that my enthusiasm for the project was contagious and that I have some cultural capital as a women's studies professor and a feminist interested in the underground world of radical menstruation. They may have seen me more as a mother figure than as a peer, but at least I was a mother they could talk to. That is, I was cool enough.

And so I dug in. I conducted preliminary fieldwork to establish the discursive and ideological frames that constitute menstrual activism. This initial fieldwork also enabled access to the network of menstrual activists and their resources. I attended the Boston Skillshare (an annual event in the local punk/DIY scene) and a menstrual health workshop on my own campus.[1] After two months, I had a breakthrough in my data collection when I connected with the Student Environmental Action Coalition (SEAC), a grassroots coalition of student and youth environmental groups. Tampaction, one of SEAC's national campaigns, was being revived after a period of abeyance. In its most recent incarnation, it endeavored to "eradicate the use of unhealthy, unsustainable tampons and pads, institutionalize sustainable alternatives into our schools and communities, and infuse healthy attitudes surrounding menstruation into our culture's consciousness. We're letting the world know that bleedin' can be everyone's issue. In doing so, we work to destroy patriarchal taboos, end environmental degradation caused by disposable tampons and pads, and promote vaginal and menstrual health."[2]

I joined the Tampaction e-mail list, which enabled me to track the hot spots for menstrual activism throughout the country and learn how individuals and small groups were enacting the Tampaction campaign in their local communities and campuses. I deepened my connection with Tampaction when I attended two of SEAC's major weekend events: their National Convergence in Boston and their Activist Training Camp at Antioch College in Yellow Springs, Ohio. Both events gave me access to dozens of menstrual activists—many of them in training—as well as to the campaign coordinators. I learned the history of and the rationale for the Tampaction campaign and participated in the train-the-trainer sessions during which activists learned how to present menstrual health and politics workshops in their local areas. I also had the pleasure of attending a Tampaction workshop geared specifically for men and enjoyed ample opportunities for informal conversations with event attendees.

After the preliminary data collection clarified my research agenda (while leaving it loose enough, of course, to be open to whatever the field presented me), I followed up with several of the attendees at these events and requested in-depth interviews. Though not everyone I invited for an interview completed one (most often, a scarcity of time was cited as the problem), the folks I met were unequivocally delighted that someone was taking an interest in what they were doing. In most cases, they gave me permission to use their actual names in my writing and speaking, and only a few requested I suppress some of their demographic information (for example, five informants did not want their sexual identity linked to their name).

At the same time I conducted interviews, I arranged visits to several campuses to observe menstrual activist work. These visits took me to geographically diverse areas, including St. Paul, Minnesota; Fort Collins, Colorado; Philadelphia and rural Pennsylvania; and rural Ohio. I also visited Elle Corazon, a shop for artisan-made goods and home of the Bloodsisters. I sorted through their menstrual gear inventory and their archives and talked into the night with one of the Bloodsisters in various hip spots around Montreal. I also observed a one-woman protest staged in honor of the thirty-fifth anniversary of the Toxic Shock Syndrome outbreak (held outside the entrance to the Society for Menstrual Cycle Research meetings in 2005), participated in a "Women's Wisdom Workshop" in Northern California (designed to "empower women to take care of their body and make informed choices about their changing cycles"), and met women in a Red Tent during the daylong Belly and Womb Conference in western Massachusetts (I attended the conference in both 2005 and 2006). In addition, I attended two screenings of Giovanna Chesler's documentary *Period. The End of Menstruation* and the lively question-and-answer sessions that followed this provocative investigation of cycle-stopping contraception.

Through these participant-observations, I recruited still more participants, whom I interviewed in depth in group settings, over the phone, or through e-mail. In every project interview, I explored the inspiration for taking on the work of menstrual activism, the tactics and strategies deployed and their effectiveness, the movements that inform menstrual activism, and the joys and challenges of doing this work (see appendix B for the interview protocol). Most interviews were with individuals, though I did conduct three group interviews. Those interviewed included artists, filmmakers, writers, midwives, campus and community organizers, cartoonists, poets, zinesters, and women's health educators. (I also interviewed two representatives from Procter & Gamble's FemCare division to hear industry responses to claims made against their product line.)[3] In all, I interviewed sixty-five activists, and I report some of the demographic information I collected about these research participants. During the final stages of the writing of the manuscript, I interviewed two influential activists with whom I had failed to connect earlier, one via e-mail. These final interviews allowed me to validate and deepen my analysis.

In the midst of my fieldwork, I, together with my research assistant Ginn Norris, reached out to alternative menstrual product makers and distributors accessed via the English-speaking World Wide Web. Our one-page questionnaire covered the demographic served, date and story of the business's founding, mission and/or vision of business, and data demonstrating business growth. Twenty-four small businesses responded, allowing me to confirm my suspicion that alternative menstrual products were indeed growing in popularity and to gain insight into the population choosing alternative products.

To round out the data necessary to construct a comprehensive understanding of menstrual activism over time, I used historical analysis, turning to key movement materials, mostly trade books (many out of print), and the historical records of the renowned Boston Women's Health Book Collective housed at the Schlesinger Library on the History of Women, which allowed me to trace the movement in its earliest, formative years. The archives, newly catalogued and a veritable treasure trove for feminist history junkies, provided a window into the tremendous effort behind the tampon safety campaign (focused primarily on standardized tampon absorbency ratings), which took at least ten years to produce results. As I've said, most of the contemporary menstrual activists I met during my research were not aware of this history—an example of the kind of blind spot feared by second-wave critics of third-wave feminism.

DATA ANALYSIS

Once all interviews were transcribed verbatim and fieldwork notes and contemporary and historical movement materials collected and organized, I began an open coding process which fractures the data, permitting me to identify salient categories and their descriptive properties.[4] Essential to this process was bracketing (as inspired by Edmund Husserl), an ethnomethodological approach that sets aside assumptions, enabling me to minimize (though surely not eliminate) my own knowledge claims from distorting the content and form of informant knowledge. Bracketing makes it more possible for informant voices to be heard. With a topic as taboo-ridden as menstruation, I found it especially important to bracket my own embodied menstrual shame, for example, when I encountered some of the bolder tactics and conceptualizations common to the menstrual activists I studied.

At the conclusion of the open coding phase, I began axial coding, "a set of procedures whereby data are put back together in new ways . . . by making connections between categories."[5] During this painstaking process, I tried to discern how the categories related to one another; considering these linkages, I constructed a conceptual framework which served to answer the most basic of empirical questions: What is going on here? And what does it mean? Through this process, I began to see not only that menstrual activism was an interesting (and little-known) movement in its own right, but also that it offered insight into the U.S. women's movement, especially third-wave feminism. The data enabled me to bring empirical texture and a more complicated rendering of the similarities and differences between the movement's second and third waves. Finally, in the tradition of participatory research, I invited two key activists to comment on my work. I shared the penultimate draft of the manuscript with a central figure in the radical menstruation wing of the movement and made several revisions based on her feedback. I also shared portions of the manuscript with an activist who was key to the feminist spiritualist wing and incorporated her challenges to my analysis as well.

Appendix B. Interview Protocol

How would you describe yourself?

What social movements, if any, do you identify with?

Do you consider yourself an activist? Why or why not?

How would you define "menstrual activism"? Do you use this language to describe what you do? Why or why not? What language do you use if different? How is this language meaningful to you?

Tell me *when* you first became interested in menstrual activism. If you can, please provide a date (or at least a year). *Who* or *what* exposed you? What was your initial reaction?

At what point did you decide to work on menstrual issues? Again, if you can, please provide an approximate date.

How did your family and friends respond to your activism? How do they respond today?

What and who are the biggest influences on your work?

What is the most rewarding aspect of being a menstrual activist? What about it makes it rewarding?

What is the most frustrating aspect of being a menstrual activist? What about it makes it frustrating?

What sort of doubts lurk around for you when you do your activism (if any)? How do you deal with them?

Tell me about a time when some activism you participated in (could be the launching of your zine or mounting of your website or the first time you held a workshop, for example) seemed a real success? Why do you think it worked?

Tell me about a "flop." Why do you think the activism failed? What did you learn from this experience?

What's the most affirming feedback you ever received about your work? How did you react to it and why?

What's the most discouraging feedback you ever received about your work? How did you react to it and why?

How would you characterize menstrual activists as a group? Is there a certain type of person that takes up this issue? A couple of different types? Can you describe the "typical" menstrual activist to me? What might account for the particular characteristics shared by menstrual activists? What makes answering this question hard or easy?

Is there a discernible community of menstrual activists? Is it a movement? Why or why not?

Where do you fit in all of this? What's your unique contribution/s?

In your opinion, what other social issues (movements, trends, initiatives) are most related to menstrual activism? What's the connection between them?

Why do you think the mainstream public remains largely uninformed about the issues you are working on (such as FemCare safety and alternatives)? What is it going to take for these issues to catch on and become more accepted?

How do you stay committed to the work you do? What's in it for you? If you have not remained active in menstrual activism, tell me what led you to move on?

What do you believe is the future of menstrual activism? Where is it headed? What's going to help it along? Slow it down?

Are there any groups that might be excluded from menstrual activism? Why might that be?

What else would you like me to know?

Appendix C. Demographics of Interviewees

(N=65)

Age	Percentage
18–22	38
23–29	20
30–45	25
45+	17
Gender identity	
Female/woman	94
Male/man	3
Gender queer	3
Economic class	
Working/poor/lower	31
Lower middle	9
Middle	38
Upper middle	20
Upper	2
Racial identity	
White	88
Latina	1
African American	5
Biracial	3
No response	3
Sexual orientation	
Heterosexual	31
Queer	63
No response	6

Appendix D. Selected Menstrual Activist Resources

Adventures in Menstruating and Chart Your Cycle
   http://www.chartyourcycle.co.uk/
Canadian Women's Health Network
   http://www.cwhn.ca/
Justisse Healthworks for Women: Fertility Awareness, Education, Natural Birth
      Control, and Holistic Reproductive Health
   http://www.justisse.ca/
MOLT: The Museum of the Menovulatory Lifetime
   http://www.moltx.org/
Moon Magic Workshop on Puberty (free curriculum available for download)
   http://www.kesakivel.com
Museum of Menstruation and Women's Health
   http://www.mum.org/
National Women's Health Network
   http://www.womenshealthnetwork.org/
Our Bodies Ourselves/The Boston Women's Health Book Collective
   http://www.ourbodiesourselves.org/
Red Tent Temple Movement
   http://alisastarkweather.com
Red Web Foundation
   http://www.redwebfoundation.org/
Scarleteen: Sex Ed for the Real World
   http://www.scarleteen.com/
Society for Menstrual Cycle Research
   http://menstruationresearch.org/
Student Environmental Action Coalition
   http://seac.org/

Notes

INTRODUCTION

1. Aimeé Darcel is adee's given name.

2. "FemCare" is the industry term for feminine care, the array of menstrual products including pads (sometimes called napkins, or, in the United Kingdom, towels), tampons, cups, and sponges.

3. A Keeper is a reusable menstrual cup made of gum rubber. Shaped like a bell with a tail, it is inserted in the vagina to collect menstrual fluid.

4. Vivien Labaton and Dawn Lundy Martin, eds., *The Fire This Time: Young Activists and the New Feminism* (New York: Anchor Books, 2004), xxi.

5. Jo Reger, introduction to *Different Wavelengths: Studies of the Contemporary Women's Movement*, ed. Jo Reger (New York: Routledge, 2005), xvi–xvii.

6. My use of the term "continuity" merits clarification. When I assert that there is continuity between the second and third waves of the U.S. women's movement, I am not implying there is direct influence (which seems to be a connotative meaning of the word). Rather, I am sticking more closely to the denotative meaning of the word—uninterrupted connection or succession. That is, because I am not prepared to discuss the various mechanisms by which third-wavers learned of second-wave tactics, I cannot make a claim that they chose to replicate the tactics I identify here, even if they, the third-wave activists, are not aware of their inspiration. Nevertheless, I find the parallels over time worthy of explanation. Finally, I do acknowledge that while similar tactics recur throughout time, they cannot be easily pinned to one source (i.e., the second wave of the U.S. women's movement). Given the cross-fertilization of movements in the same era, it is nearly impossible to establish who (or what) initiated a particular tactic.

7. For examples of personal narrative, see Kathy Bail, ed., *DIY Feminism* (St. Leonards, NSW, Australia: Allen and Unwin, 1996); Veronica Chambers, *Mama's Girl* (New York: Riverhead, 1996); Barbara Findlen, ed., *Listen Up! Voices from the Next Feminist Generation*, 2nd ed. (Seattle: Seal Press, 2001); Labaton and Martin, *The Fire This Time*; Daisy Hernández and Bushra Rehman, eds., *Colonize This! Young Women of Color on Today's Feminism* (Seattle: Seal Press, 2002); Lisa Jones, *Bulletproof Diva: Tales of Race, Sex, and Hair* (New York: Doubleday, 1994); Joan Morgan, *When Chickenheads Come*

Home to Roost: My Life as a Hip-Hop Feminist (New York: Simon and Schuster, 1999); Rory Dicker and Alison Piepmeier, eds., *Catching a Wave: Reclaiming Feminism for the 21st Century* (Boston: Northeastern University Press, 2003); Rebecca Walker, "Becoming the Third Wave," in *Testimony: Young African Americans on Self-Discovery and Black Identity*, ed. Natasha Tarpley (Boston: Beacon Press, 1995). Scholarly treatments include, for example, Stacey Gillis, Gillian Howie, and Rebecca Munford, *Third Wave Feminism: A Critical Exploration*, 2nd ed. (New York: Palgrave Macmillan, 2007); Astrid Henry, *Not My Mother's Sister: Generational Conflict and Third-Wave Feminism* (Bloomington: Indiana University Press, 2004); Leslie Heywood and Jennifer Drake, eds., *Third-Wave Agenda: Being Feminist, Doing Feminism* (Minneapolis: University of Minnesota Press, 1997); Catherine Orr, "Charting the Currents of the Third Wave," *Hypatia* 12 (1997): 29–45; Kimberly Springer, "Third-Wave Black Feminism?" *Signs: Journal of Women in Culture and Society* 27, no. 4 (2002): 1059–1082.

8. While I acknowledge the uneasiness surrounding the term "third wave," it remains the dominant language used to describe the newest iteration of the women's movement. Thus, unless a particular writer or organization uses different terminology in their self-identification, I use the label "third wave."

9. Labaton and Martin, *The Fire This Time*, xxv.

10. Henry, *Not My Mother's Sister*, 11.

11. *Don't Let the System Get You Done: Cheer Up!* DVD, directed and produced by Jen Nedbalsky and Mary Christmas (New York, NYC Radical Cheerleaders, 2004).

12. Natalie Fixmer and Julia Wood, "The Personal Is Still Political: Embodied Politics in Third Wave Feminism," *Women's Studies in Communication* 28, no. 2 (2005): 235–257.

13. Gina Bellafante, "It's All About Me!" *Time*, June 29, 1998.

14. Susan Brownmiller, *In Our Time: Memoir of a Revolution* (New York: Dial Press, 1999), 62.

15. Leila Rupp, *Worlds of Women: The Making of an International Women's Movement* (Princeton, N.J.: Princeton University Press, 1997), 62.

16. Springer, "Third-Wave Black Feminism?" 1061.

17. Nancy Naples, "Confronting the Future, Learning from the Past: Feminist Praxis in the Twenty-first Century," in *Different Wavelengths*, ed. Reger, 224, 218; Nancy Whittier, *Feminist Generations: The Persistence of the Radical Women's Movement* (Philadelphia: Temple University Press, 1995).

18. Lisa Jervis, "Goodbye to Feminism's Generational Divide," in *We Don't Need Another Wave*, ed. Melody Berger (Emeryville, Calif.: Seal Press, 2006), 14.

19. Looser qtd. in Henry, *Not My Mother's Sister*, 12.

20. Henry, *Not My Mother's Sister*. I thank Liz Kissling for enriching my thinking about the multiple problems with the mother-daughter trope.

21. For example, see Reger, *Different Wavelengths*; Whittier, *Feminist Generations*.

22. On cultural attitudes about the menstrual cycle, see, for example, Jane Delaney, Mary Jane Lupton, and Emily Toth, *The Curse: A Cultural History of Menstruation* (New York: Dutton, 1976); Sharon Golub, ed., *Lifting the Curse of Menstruation: A Feminist Appraisal of the Influence of Menstruation on Women's Lives* (New York: Harrington Park Press, 1985); Sophie Laws, *Issues of Blood: The Politics of Menstruation* (New York: Macmillan, 1990); Jane Ussher, *Managing the Monstrous Feminine: Regulating the Reproductive Body* (New York: Routledge, 2006); Janet Lee, "Menarche and the (Hetero) Sexualization of the Female Body," in *The Politics of Women's Bodies: Sexuality, Appearance, and Behavior*, ed. Rose Weitz (Oxford: Oxford University Press, 2003),

82–89. For rhetorical analyses of media representations of menstruation and related products, see, for example, Mindy Erchull, Joan Chrisler, Jennifer Gorman, and Ingrid Johnston-Robledo, "Education and Advertising: A Content Analysis of Commercially Produced Booklets about Menstruation," *Journal of Early Adolescence* 22, no. 4 (2002); Ingrid Johnston-Robledo, Jessica Barnack, and Stephanie Wares, "Kiss Your Period Good-Bye: Menstrual Suppression in the Popular Press," *Sex Roles* 54 (2006): 353–360; Elizabeth Kissling, *Capitalizing on the Curse: The Business of Menstruation* (Boulder, Colo.: Lynne Reiner, 2006); David Linton, "The Media and Menstruation: Images and Public Relations," paper presented at the National Communication Association Annual Conference, November 22, 2003, Miami Beach, Fla.

23. For example, see Susan Bordo and Allison Jaggar, eds., *Gender/Body/Knowledge* (New Brunswick, N.J.: Rutgers University Press, 1989); Judith Butler, *Bodies That Matter: On the Discursive Limits of Sex* (New York: Routledge, 1993); Kate Conboy, Nadia Medina, and Sarah Stanbury, eds., *Writing on the Body: Female Embodiment and Feminist Theory* (New York: Columbia University Press, 1997); Emily Martin, *The Woman in the Body: A Cultural Analysis of Reproduction*, rev. ed. (Boston: Beacon Press, 2001); Rose Weitz, ed., *The Politics of Women's Bodies: Sexuality, Appearance, and Behavior*, 2nd ed. (Oxford: Oxford University Press, 2003).

24. Joan Jacobs Brumberg, *The Body Project: An Intimate History of American Girls* (New York: Vintage Books, 1997), 32.

25. Seasonale and Lybrel are both oral contraceptives. But unlike standard birth-control pills, which are taken for three weeks followed by a week of placebos (during the latter, women experience what's called a "withdrawal bleed" [not an actual period]), these pills are taken continuously and thus suppress menstruation. Seasonale (made by Barr Laboratories) suppresses all but four withdrawal bleeds in a calendar year; Lybrel (made by Wyeth) eliminates withdrawal bleeding completely.

26. Linda Andrist, Alex Hoyt, Dawn Weinstein, and Chris McGibbon, "The Need to Bleed: Women's Attitudes and Beliefs about Menstrual Suppression," *Journal of the American Academy of Nurse Practitioners* 16, no. 1 (2004): 36.

27. Karen Houppert, *The Curse: Confronting the Last Unmentionable Taboo: Menstruation* (New York: Farrar, Strauss and Giroux, 1999), 13.

28. See Morgan, *When Chickenheads Come Home to Roost*; Sheryl Ruzek, *The Women's Health Movement: Feminist Alternatives to Medical Control* (New York: Praeger, 1979); Carol Weisman, *Women's Health Care: Activist Traditions and Institutional Change* (Baltimore: Johns Hopkins University Press, 1998); Mary Zimmerman, "The Women's Health Movement: A Critique of the Medical Enterprise and the Position of Women," in *Analyzing Gender: A Handbook of Social Science Research*, ed. B. Hess and M. M. Ferree (Newbury Park, Calif.: Sage, 1987).

29. While my choice of the word "wings" was not intended as a menstrual product pun, I acknowledge the humor. Thanks to Liz Kissling, who playfully made this obvious.

30. Michelle Meadows, "Tampon Safety: TSS Now Rare, but Women Should Still Take Care," http://www.fda.gov/fdac/features/2000/200 tss.html (accessed March 24, 2008).

31. Philip Tierno, *The Secret Life of Germs: What They Are, Why We Need Them, and How We Can Protect Ourselves against Them* (New York: Atria Books, 2001), 75.

32. In the sense that radical menstruation activists call for an end to capitalism as we know it and in their modest DIY way practice and promote a means to slowly erode capitalism's power, I consider their activism both radical and revolutionary. Admittedly, such actions are not comparable to the revolutionary tactics of infamous groups like the

radical left group the Weathermen, who demanded the overthrow of the U.S. government and the destruction of the capitalist system.

33. Bloodsisters, "At Once Old and New," *Collective Red Alert #3* (1996), 3. Reprinted with permission.

34. Naples, "Confronting the Future," 222.

35. For example, see Hernández and Rehman, *Colonize This!*

36. Wini Breines, *The Trouble between Us: An Uneasy History of White and Black Women in the Feminist Movement* (Oxford: Oxford University Press, 2006).

37. On the marginalizing of women of color, see, for example, Cherrie Moraga and Gloria Anzaldùa, eds., *This Bridge Called My Back: Writings by Radical Women of Color* (New York: Kitchen Table/Women of Color Press, 1983).

38. Evelyn Brooks Higginbotham, *Righteous Discontent: The Women's Movement in the Black Baptist Church,* 1880–1920 (Cambridge, Mass.: Harvard University Press, 1993).

39. "Genderqueer" describes a person who identifies as neither man nor woman. Genderqueer persons may locate their gender identity somewhere *between* man and woman or as *both* man and woman, or they may reject gender identity altogether. See, for example, Joan Nestle, Clare Howell, and Riki Wilchins, eds., *GenderQueer: Voices from Beyond the Sexual Binary* (Los Angeles: Alyson Books, 2002).

40. The phrase "living Butler" denotes the practical application of key ideas associated with celebrated feminist theorist Judith Butler: the intentional development and deployment of activist agendas, including tactical approaches and linguistic choices, that refuse to subscribe to the gender binary. I am indebted to Christine Cooper for alerting me to this point. The phrase "living Butler" is hers.

41. Nancy Whittier, "From the Second to the Third Wave: Continuity and Change in Grassroots Feminism," in *The U.S. Women's Movement in Global Perspective: People, Passions, and Power,* ed. Lee Ann Banaszak (Lanham, Md.: Rowman and Littlefield, 2006), 45–67.

1 — ENCOUNTERING THIRD-WAVE FEMINISM

1. U.S. Senate Committee on the Judiciary: S. Hrg. 102–1084, Pt. 4, Hearings on the Nomination of Clarence Thomas to be Associate Justice of the Supreme Court October 11, 1991, http://www.gpoaccess.gov/congress/senate/judiciary/sh102–1084pt4/ browse.html (accessed September 9, 2009).

2. Walker, "Becoming the Third Wave," 216. This reference points to a reprinting of Walker's essay in Natasha Tarpley's edited anthology *Testimony: Young African Americans on Self-Discovery and Black Identity.*

3. Reger, *Different Wavelengths,* xxiii; Lynn Chancer, *Reconcilable Differences: Confronting Beauty, Pornography, and the Future of Feminism* (Berkeley: University of California Press, 1998), 265.

4. Henry, *Not My Mothers Sister,* 23. See Deborah Rosenfelt and Judith Stacey, "Second Thoughts on the Second Wave," *Feminist Review* 27 (1987): 359. Curiously, the structural, macro, policy-level issues Rosenfelt and Stacey mention—pay equity, child care, maternal and child health, work schedules, and parental leave—are not the issues that have emerged as central to third-wave feminism.

5. Naomi Wolf, *Fire with Fire: The New Female Power and How It Will Change the 21st Century* (New York, Random House, 1993).

6. The 3rdWWWave: Feminism for the New Millennium, http://www.3rdwwwave.com (accessed June 29, 2007).

7. Heywood and Drake, *Third-Wave Agenda*, 9.

8. Jennifer Baumgardner and Amy Richards, *Manifesta: Young Women, Feminism, and the Future* (New York: Farrar, Strauss and Giroux, 2000), 15.

9. Heywood and Drake, *Third-Wave Agenda*, 4.

10. Dicker and Piepmeier, *Catching a Wave*, 14.

11. Henry, *Not My Mother's Sister*, 3.

12. Ibid., 5, 12.

13. Judith Lorber, *Gender Inequality: Feminist Theories and Politics*, 3rd ed. (Los Angeles: Roxbury, 2005), 279.

14. Gillis, Howie, and Munford, *Third Wave Feminism*, 3; Amber Kinser, ed., *Mothering in the Third Wave* (Toronto: Demeter Press, 2007); Springer, "Third-Wave Black Feminism?"

15. Reger, *Different Wavelengths*, xvii.

16. The writers of these texts cannot be easily categorized. They come from a wide array of racial, ethnic, and class backgrounds and claim a variety of sexual orientations, though most are urban, college-educated women under thirty-five.

17. Rebecca Walker, introduction to *To Be Real: Telling the Truth and Changing the Face of Feminism*, ed. Walker (New York: Anchor Books, 1995), xxxiv; Anastasia Higginbotham, "Chicks Goin' At It," in *Listen Up!* ed. Findlen, 17; Lisa Weiner-Mahfuz, "Organizing 101: A Mixed-Race Feminist in Movements for Social Justice," in *Colonize This!* ed. Hernández and Rehman, 39.

18. See Susan Muaddi Darraj, "It's Not an Oxymoron: The Search for Arab Feminism," in *Colonize This!* ed. Hernández and Rehman, 295–311; Sonja Curry-Johnson, "Weaving an Identity Tapestry," in *Listen Up!* ed. Findlen, 221–229.

19. Pandora Leong, "Living outside the Box," in *Colonize This!* ed. Hernández and Rehman, 353.

20. Anna Bondoc, "Close But No Banana," in *To Be Real*, ed. Walker, 184.

21. On Truth's speech, see, for instance, Eleanor Flexner, *Century of Struggle: The Women's Rights Movement in the United States* (Cambridge, Mass.: Belknap Press, 1975), 91; on Brown's statement, see Alice Echols, *Daring to Be Bad: Radical Feminism in America, 1967–1975* (Minneapolis: University of Minnesota Press, 1989), 213.

22. Nomy Lamm, "It's a Big Fat Revolution," in *Listen Up!* ed. Findlen, 55.

23. Orr, "Charting the Currents of the Third Wave."

24. Labaton and Martin, *The Fire This Time*, xxi. For example, see Joshua Breitbart and Ana Nogueira, "An Independent Media Center of One's Own: A Feminist Alternative to Corporate Media," in ibid., 19–41.

25. Jean Mocha Herrup, "Virtual Identity," in *To Be Real*, ed. Walker, 247.

26. Lorde qtd. in Labaton and Martin, *The Fire This Time*, 285; ibid., xxvi; Curry-Johnson, "Weaving an Identity Tapestry," 53; Danzy Senna, "To Be Real," in *To Be Real*, ed. Walker, 16.

27. Patricia Hill Collins, *Black Feminist Thought: Knowledge, Consciousness and the Politics of Empowerment* (New York: Routledge, 2000), 227–228.

28. "A Black Feminist Statement by the Combahee River Collective," Feminist eZine, http://www.feministezine.com/feminist/modern/ Black-Feminist-Statement.html (accessed July 29, 2007).

29. Cristina Tzintzún, "Colonize This," in *Colonize This!* ed. Hernández and Rehman, 28; Walker, introduction, xxxv; Christine Doza, "Bloodlove," in *Listen Up!* ed. Findlen, 43.

30. Naples, "Confronting the Future," 227; Gillis, Howie, and Munford, *Third Wave Feminism*, xxi, emphasis in original.

31. Orr, *Hypatia*, 37.

32. Baumgardner and Richards, *Manifesta*, xi.

33. Siobhan Brooks, "Black Feminism in Everyday Life: Race, Mental Illness, Poverty, and Motherhood," in *Colonize This!* ed. Hernández and Rehman, 116; Kiini Ibura Salaam, "How Sexual Harassment Slaughtered, Then Saved Me," in ibid., 328.

34. Lamm, "It's a Big Fat Revolution," 134; Cecilia Balli, "Thirty Eight," in *Colonize This!* ed. Hernández and Rehman, 197.

35. JeeYeun Lee, "Beyond Bean Counting," in *Listen Up!* ed. Findlen, 69.

36. Baumgardner and Richards, *Manifesta*, 80; Reger, *Different Wavelengths*, xxi.

37. Lisa Hogeland, "Against Generational Thinking, or Something That 'Third-Wave' Feminism Isn't," *Women's Studies in Communication* 24 (2001): 115.

38. Orr, *Hypatia*, 32.

39. For example, Winifred Breines, *The Trouble between Us: An Uneasy History of White and Black Women in the Feminist Movement* (New York: Oxford University Press, 2006); Flora Davis, *Moving the Mountain: The Women's Movement in America, since 1960* (Urbana: University of Illinois, 1999); Rachel Blau DuPlessis and Ann Snitow, eds., *The Feminist Memoir Project: Voices from Women's Liberation* (New York: Three Rivers Press, 1998); Echols, *Daring to Be Bad*; Ruth Rosen, *The World Split Open: How the Modern Women's Movement Changed America* (New York: Viking, 2000); Benita Roth, *Separate Roads to Feminism: Black, Chicana, and White Feminist Movements in America's Second-Wave* (Cambridge: Cambridge University Press, 2004); and Barbara Ryan, *Feminism and the Women's Movement: Dynamics of Change in Social Movement Ideology and Activism* (New York: Praeger, 1979).

40. Reger, *Different Wavelengths*, xxi.

41. For more information, see Dexter Bloomer, *Life and Writings of Amelia Bloomer* (New York: Schocken Books, 1975).

42. Gloria Steinem, foreword," in *To Be Real*, ed. Walker, xxii; Dicker and Piepmeier, *Catching a Wave*, 14–15.

43. Kimberly Springer, "Third-Wave Black Feminism?" *Signs: Journal of Women in Culture and Society* 27, no. 4 (2002): 1059–1082.

44. Henry, *Not My Mother's Sister*, 2–3.

45. See Barry Adam, *The Rise of a Gay and Lesbian Movement* (Boston: Twayne, 1987); Douglas Crimp, *AIDS: Cultural Analysis/Cultural Activism* (Cambridge, Mass.: MIT Press, 1998); Eric Marcus, *Making Gay History: The Half-Century Fight for Lesbian and Gay Rights* (New York: Harper, 2002).

46. Joshua Gamson, "Must Identity Movements Self-Destruct? A Queer Dilemma," in *American Queer: Now and Then*, ed. David Schneer and Caryn Aviv (Boulder, Colo.: Paradigm, 2006), 254. I thank Jean Humez for pointing out the similarities in intramovement struggle across social movements.

47. Reger, *Different Wavelengths*, xxi.

48. Adrienne Rich, *Of Woman Born: Motherhood as Experience and Institution* (New York: Bantam, 1977), 254.

2 — FEMINIST ENGAGEMENTS WITH MENSTRUATION

1. Cynthia Enloe, *The Curious Feminist: Searching for Women in a New Age of Empire* (Berkeley: University of California Press, 2004), 3.

2. Houppert, *The Curse*, 13–47; Kissling, *Capitalizing on the Curse*, 4; Alice Dan and Linda Lewis, eds., *Menstrual Health in Women's Lives* (Urbana: University of Illinois Press, 1992), 1.

3. Arika Okrent, *In the Land of Invented Languages: Esperanto Rock Stars, Klingon Poets, Logian Lovers, and the Mad Dreamers Who Tried to Build a Perfect Language* (New York: Spiegel and Grau, 2009), 243–244.

4. Alice J. Dan, "What Have We Learned? An Historical View of the Society for Menstrual Cycle Research," *NSWA Journal* 16, no. 3 (2004): 45.

5. Laura Fingerson, *Girls in Power: Gender, Body, and Menstruation in Adolescence* (Albany: State University of New York Press, 2006), 4.

6. Thomas Buckley and Alma Gottlieb, eds., *Blood Magic: The Anthropology of Menstruation* (Berkeley: University of California Press, 1988); Chris Knight, *Blood Relations: Menstruation and the Origins of Culture* (New Haven: Yale University Press, 1991); Penelope Shuttle and Peter Redgrove, *The Wise Wound: Myths, Realities, and Meanings of Menstruation* (New York: Bantam Books, 1990).

7. Laws, *Issues of Blood*, 211.

8. Evelyn Brooks Higginbotham, *Righteous Discontent: The Women's Movement in the Black Baptist Church*, 1880–1920 (Cambridge, Mass.: Harvard University Press, 1993). I explore this concept in some detail in chapter 6.

9. Elizabeth Grosz, "Sexual Difference and the Problem of Essentialism," in *The Essential Difference*, ed. Naomi Schor and Elizabeth Weed (Bloomington: Indiana University Press, 1994), 203.

10. Beausang qtd. in Maria Luisa Marván, Claudia Morales, and Sandra Cortés-Iniestra, "Emotional Reactions to Menarche among Mexican Women of Different Generations," *Sex Roles* 54 (2006): 324.

11. See Marván, Morales, and Cortés-Iniestra, "Emotional Reactions"; and Britt-Marie Thurén, "'Opening Doors and Getting Rid of Shame': Experiences of First Menstruation in Valencia, Spain," *Women's Studies International* 17 (1994), 217–228, for example.

12. Marván, Morales, and Cortés-Iniestra, "Emotional Reactions," 323–330.

13. Ayse Uskul, "Women's Menarche Stories from a Multicultural Sample," *Social Science and Medicine* 59 (2004): 667–679.

14. John McMaster, Kenna Cormie, and Marian Pitts, "Menstrual and Premenstrual Experiences of Women in a Developing Country," *Health Care for Women International* 18 (1997): 533–541.

15. Catherine So-Kum Tang, Dannii Yuen-Lan Yeung, and Antyoinette Marie Lee, "Psychosocial Correlates of Emotional Responses to Menarche among Chinese Adolescent Girls," *Journal of Adolescent Health* 33 (2003): 193–201

16. Ros Bramwell, "Blood and Milk: Constructions of Female Bodily Fluids in Western Society," in *Women's Health: Readings on Social, Economic and Political Issues*, ed. Nancy Worcester and Mariamne Whatley (Dubuque, Iowa: Kendall/Hunt, 2004), 511–512.

17. Here and throughout this book, I use the word "taboo" to refer to that which is forbidden, prohibited, or discouraged in discourses, representations, and explicit practices due to sociocultural value systems that render the subject in question socially unacceptable

18. For classical Greece, see Etienne Van De Walle and Elisha Renne, eds., *Regulating Menstruation: Beliefs, Practices, Interpretations* (Chicago: University of Chicago Press, 2001), xix; Leviticus 15:19, *Holy Bible New Revised Standard Version, Classic* (Nashville: Abingdon Press, 2009).

19. Martin, *The Woman in the Body*, 31.

20. Joan Jacobs Brumberg, *The Body Project: An Intimate History of American Girls* (New York: Vintage, 1998), 30. In chapter 4, I critically engage this particular framing of menstruation.

21. Andrew Shail and Gillian Howie, "'Talking Your Body's Language': The Menstrual Materialisations of Sexed Ontology," in *Menstruation: A Cultural History*, ed. Shail and Howie (New York: Palgrave Macmillan, 2005), 1–2; Brumberg, *The Body Project*, 55.

22. Michel Foucault, *Discipline and Punish: The Birth of a Prison*, 2nd ed., trans. Alan Sheridan (New York: Vintage Books, 1990).

23. As Susan Bordo stresses in *Unbearable Weight: Feminism, Western Culture, and the Body* (Berkeley: University of California Press, 1993), although Foucault is most often associated with the theorizing of the body as disciplined, formulations of the body as a political site are largely the contribution of feminist thinking that dates as far back as Mary Wollstonecraft, who articulated the social construction of (privileged) femininity as docility in the late eighteenth century (17–18).

24. Foucault, *Discipline and Punish*, 201.

25. Sandra Lee Bartky, *Femininity and Domination: Studies in the Phenomenology of Oppression* (New York: Routledge, 1990), 65.

26. Monique Deveaux, "Feminism and Empowerment: A Critical Reading of Foucault," in *Feminist Approaches in Theory and Methodology: An Interdisciplinary Reader*, ed. Sharlene Hesse-Biber, Christina Gilmartin, and Robin Lyndenberg (New York: Oxford University Press, 1999), 236, 239.

27. Martin, *The Woman in the Body*, 46. Applying a gender lens to her analysis, Martin elaborates: "Perhaps one reason the negative image of failed production is attached to menstruation is precisely that women are in some sinister sense out of control when they menstruate. They are not reproducing, not continuing the species, not preparing to stay at home with the baby, not providing a safe, warm womb to nurture a man's sperm" (47).

28. Thomas Laqueur, *Making Sex: Body and Gender from the Greeks to Freud* (Cambridge, Mass.: Harvard University Press, 1990), 221, 210.

29. Martin, *The Woman in the Body*, 52–53.

30. Louise Lander, *Images of Bleeding: Menstruation as Ideology* (New York: Orlando Press, 1988), 1–2. Thanks to careful reader Jean Humez for calling my attention to this implication.

31. In response to President Barack Obama's nomination of now Supreme Court Justice Sonia Sotomayor to the Court, conservative radio talk-show host G. Gordon Liddy quipped: "Let's hope that the key conferences aren't when she's menstruating or something, or just before she's going to menstruate. That would really be bad. Lord knows what we would get then." *The G. Gordon Liddy Show*, Radio America, May 28, 2009.

32. Lander, *Images of Bleeding*, 5.

33. Golub, *Lifting the Curse of Menstruation*, xii.

34. Kissling, *Capitalizing on the Curse*, 38, 39.

35. Diana Taylor, *Taking Back the Month: A Personalized Solution for Managing PMS and Enhancing Your Health* (New York: Perigee, 2002); Linaya Hahn, *PMS—Solving the Puzzle: 16 Causes of PMS and What to Do about It!* (Evanston, Ill.: Spectrum Press, 1995); Stephanie DeGraff Bender and Kathleen Kelleher, *PMS: Women Tell Women How to Control Premenstrual Syndrome* (Oakland, CA: New Harbinger Publications, 1996); Stephanie DeGraff Bender and Kathleen Kelleher, *PMS: A Positive Program to Gain Control* (Tucson, Ariz.: Body Press, 1986); Katharina Dalton and Wendy Holton, *Once a Month: Understanding and Treating PMS* (Alameda, Calif.: Hunter House, 1999); *Vinnie's Cramp-Kicking Remedies: And Other Clever Cures for PMS, Bloating, and More* (San Francisco: Chronicle Books, 2004); Joseph Martorano and Maureen Morgan, *Unmasking PMS: The Complete PMS Medical Treatment Plan* (New York: M. Evans, 1993).

36. Lander, *Images of Bleeding*, 100.

37. Ibid., 101.

38. Kissling, *Capitalizing on the Curse*, 50.

39. Here, I am implying that because many people feel compelled to hide or minimize their mental illness, such as clinical depression, treatment for PMDD is intentionally dissociated from treatment for depression.

40. Gadsby qtd. in Kissling, *Capitalizing on the Curse*, 50–51.

41. Ibid., 55.

42. For a cycle-stopping contraception campaign masked as a public information resource, see PeriodsLessOften, http://www.periodslessoften.ca/. The website is operated by an anonymous "research-based pharmaceutical company."

43. "Menstruation Is Not a Disease," Society for Menstrual Cycle Research, http://menstruationresearch.org/position/menstrual-suppression-new-2007/ (accessed August 17, 2007). In the interest of full disclosure, I serve on the board of this organization and was among several board members who drafted and edited this statement.

44. Johnston-Robledo, Barnack, and Wares, "'Kiss Your Period Good-bye,'" 16, 18.

45. Martin, *The Woman in the Body*, xiv, xvi

46. Andrist et al., "The Need to Bleed," 4.

47. Some, like physician and author Susan Rako, author of *No More Periods? The Risks of Menstrual Suppression and Other Cutting-Edge Issues about Hormones and Women's Health* (New York: Harmony Books, 2003), raised the (red) flag of concerns associated with continuous-use contraception. Osteoporosis, heart attacks, strokes, cancer, and heart problems, she claims, are all potential risks faced by women who use extended-cycle oral birth control to suppress menstruation. In a nutshell, Rako's argument is that the natural menstrual cycle lowers blood pressure (for half the cycle), reduces a woman's iron stores, and links to "every organ system in the body" (31). Thus, constant dosing with estrogen compromises key regulating functions. In other words, the menstrual cycle is more than a monthly shedding of the uterine lining; the ebb and flow of a woman's hormones are essential to her overall health and well-being. Press coverage of cycle-suppressing contraception never discusses these functions of the menstrual cycle. See Johnson-Robledo, Barnack, and Wares, "Kiss Your Period Good-bye."

48. See, on cesarean sections, Katherine Beckett, "Choosing Cesarean: Feminism and the Politics of Childbirth in the United States," *Feminist Theory* 6: 3 (2005): 251–275; on surrogate motherhood, Laura Purdy, *Reproducing Persons: Issues in Feminist Bioethics* (Ithaca, N.Y.: Cornell University Press, 1996); on plastic surgery, Kathy Davis, *Reshaping the Female Body: The Dilemma of Cosmetic Surgery* (New York: Routledge, 1995), and Victoria Pitts, *Surgery Junkies: The Cultural Boundaries of Cosmetic Surgery* (New Brunswick, N.J.: Rutgers University Press, 2007)

49. Cheryl Miller, "Blood, Spite, and Fears: The Strange Feminist Reaction to Lybrel," *Reason*, http://www.reason.com/news/show/119900.html (accessed August 17, 2007), 1, 2; Society for Menstrual Cycle Research, "Menstrual Suppression," SMCR Meeting, Vancouver, B.C., June 2007, http://menstruationresearch.org/position/menstrual-suppression-new-2007/ (accessed August 17, 2007).

50. Margaret Morganroth Gullette, *Aged by Culture* (Chicago: University of Chicago Press, 2004), 29. Menopause occurs when the ovaries stop producing estrogen. During this transition, which typically lasts one year, symptoms such as hot flashes, heart palpitations, vaginal dryness, and emotional distress—including mood swings, depression, anxiety, and irritability—can appear. Some women report a loss of concentration. The

decrease in estrogen production carries some risks, most significantly of osteoporosis and heart disease. Because the symptoms associated with menopause and the risks associated with postmenopause are a concern for many women, some seek medical intervention.

51. Boston Women's Health Book Collective, *Our Bodies, Ourselves: A New Edition for a New Era* (New York: Simon and Schuster, 2005), 538. HRT, a misnomer, implies that the drop in a menopausal woman's hormone levels is necessarily problematic and necessitates intervention. In 2001, the Society for Menstrual Cycle Research adopted a resolution stating: "Whereas menopause is a normal phase of every woman's life and not an estrogen deficiency condition, the term 'Hormone Replacement Therapy (HRT)' should no longer be used." The SMCR prescribes the term "Ovarian Hormone Therapy (OHT)" to refer to menopausal treatment with estrogen or progesterone. Society for Menstrual Cycle Research Blog, http://menstruationresearch.org/position/womens-health-initiative-hrt/ (accessed June 11, 2009).

52. National Women's Health Network, "Menopause Hormone Therapy Overview," http://www.nwhn.org/news/fact_sheets?story=18 (accessed August 17, 2007).

53. Martin, *The Woman in the Body*, 42, 45; Boston Women's Health Book Collective, *Our Bodies, Ourselves: A New Edition*, 538–539.

54. Brumberg, *The Body Project*, 55.

3 — THE EMERGENCE OF MENSTRUAL ACTIVISM

1. "Deb" is a pseudonym. In 1979 Jeannine Parvati published *Hygieia: A Woman's Herbal* (Monroe, Utah: Freestone Publishing Collective, 1979). It is described on its back cover as "the first book of its kind to interweave the ancient practice of herbalism with the new women's consciousness and holistic health."

2. Zimmerman, "The Women's Health Movement," 443. See also Nancy Fatt, "Women's Occupational Health and the Women's Health Movement," *Preventative Medicine* 7, no. 3 (1978): 366–371; Helen Marieskind, "The Women's Health Movement," *International Journal of Health Services* 5, no. 2 (1975): 217–223; Sandra Morgen, *Into Our Own Hands* (New Brunswick, N.J.: Rutgers University Press, 2002); Ruzek, *The Women's Health Movement*; Weisman, *Women's Health Care*.

3. Ruzek, *The Women's Health Movement*, 222.

4. Morgen, *Into Our Own Hands*, 5.

5. Qtd. in Lauria Joe, "Barbara Seaman: Muckraker for Women's Health," *Women's eNews* (October 2003), under "Journalist of the Month," http://www.womensenews.org/article.cfm?aid=1566 (accessed August 20, 2007).

6. "Our Bodies, Ourselves Timeline," http://www.ourbodiesourselves.org/about/timeline.asp (accessed June 9, 2009).

7. For example, see Brownmiller, *In Our Time*; Morgen, *Into Our Own Hands*; Ruzek, *The Women's Health Movement*.

8. See Barbara Brehm, "Knowledge Is Power: *Our Bodies, Ourselves* and the Boston Women's Health Book Collective," in *Women on Power: Leadership Redefined*, ed. Sue Freeman, Susan Bourque, and Christine Shelton (Boston: Northeastern University Press, 2001); Marianne McPherson, "Blood, Breasts, and the Royal V: Challenges of Revising Anatomy and Periods for the 2005 Edition of *Our Bodies, Ourselves*," *NWSA Journal* 17, no. 1 (2005): 190. For more discussion regarding the production of the newest *OBOS*, released spring 2005, see Heather Stephenson, "*Our Bodies, Ourselves* for a New Generation: Revising a Feminist Classic," *NWSA Journal* 27, no. 1 (2005), 173–174. Zobeida Bonilla,

"Including Every Woman: The All-Embracing 'We' of *Our Bodies, Ourselves*," *NWSA Journal* 17, no. 1 (2005), 175–183; Elizabeth Sarah Lindsey, "Reexamining Gender and Sexual Orientation: Revisioning the Representation of Queer and Trans People in the 2005 Edition of *Our Bodies, Ourselves*," *NWSA Journal* 17, no. 1 (2005), 184–189. I served as a reviewer of the chapter on reproduction, anatomy, and the menstrual cycle of the 2005 edition of *OBOS* and contributed a one-page article titled "Menstrual Activism" (253).

9. Robert Mayer, *The Consumer Movement: Guardians of the Marketplace* (Boston: Twayne, 1989), 1, 31, 375.

10. Ibid., 30.

11. Mark Dowie, *Losing Ground: American Environmentalism at the Close of the Twentieth Century* (Cambridge, Mass.: MIT Press, 1995), 3.

12. Ibid., xiii.

13. Greta Gaard, ed., *Ecofeminism: Women, Animals, Nature* (Philadelphia: Temple University Press, 1993), 3.

14. Echols, *Daring to Be Bad*, 93.

15. Judy Chicago, *Through the Flower: My Struggle as a Woman Artist* (New York: Authors Choice, 2006), 136; Edward Lucie-Smith and Judy Chicago, *Judy Chicago: An American Vision* (New York: Watson-Guptill Publications, 2000), 28.

16. Brumberg, *The Body Project*, 31.

17. Boston Women's Health Book Collective, *Our Bodies, Ourselves: A Book by and for Women* (New York: Simon and Schuster, 1973), 19.

18. Again, the environmental consequences of such disposable or single-use products were not addressed. The U.S. environmental movement—newly transitioning from its historic interest in preserving lands for recreation and pleasure to a movement more broadly conceived—did not yet register the environmental degradation associated with menstrual products.

19. For more on menstrual extraction as feminist self-help, see Denise Copelton, "Menstrual Extraction, Abortion, and the Political Context of Feminist Self-Help," in *Advances in Gender Research—Gender Perspectives on Reproduction and Sexuality*, ed. M. T. Segal, V. Demos, and J. J. Kronenfeld (London: Elsevier, 2004), 8; Ruzek, *The Women's Health Movement*; Federation of Feminist Women's Health Centers, *A New View of a Woman's Body*, 2nd ed. (Los Angeles: Feminist Health Press, 1995); Boston Women's Health Book Collective, *Our Bodies, Ourselves: A Book by and for Women* (New York: Simon and Schuster, 1973), 19.

20. Emily Culpepper, "Menstruation Consciousness Raising: A Personal and Pedagogical Process," in *Menstrual Health in Women's Lives*, ed. Dan and Lewis, 275.

21. Demonstrating the tenacity of this view of Culpepper's expertise (and the way a renegade project becomes a classic), *Period Piece* was shown at the Harvard Divinity School in 2005 in celebration of the film's groundbreaking impact. In 2006, the film was made available on DVD.

22. According to Harry Finley, curator of the online Museum of Menstruation, the Anna Health Sponge was the first sea sponge marketed as an alternative tampon; Finley hypothesizes that the product was introduced in the 1940s. http://www.mum.org/sponge2.htm.

23. *Menses*, in DVD collection *Dyketactics and Other Films from the 1970s*, directed and produced by Barbara Hammer (1974).

24. Delaney, Lupton, and Toth, *The Curse*, 222.

25. Ibid., 224.

26. For example, see Susan Perry and Jim Dawson, *Nightmare: Women and the Dalkon Shield* (New York: Macmillan, 1985).

27. Paula Weideger, *Menstruation and Menopause: The Physiology and Psychology, the Myth and the Reality*. New York: Knopf. 1976.

28. Delaney, Lupton, and Toth, *The Curse*, 110, 111. The assumption of powerlessness ("such reports will probably have no effect") is not shared by the activists who author the material on menstruation for *OBOS*, who actively engage the FDA and other government entities, as well as the FemCare industry itself, to press for menstrual product safety.

29. Ibid., 114, 113.

30. "Women's Movement under Siege," *Time*, September 26, 1977, http://www.time .com/time/magazine/article/0,9171,879788,00.html (accessed August 21, 2007).

31. Norma Swenson, "Eulogy in Memory of Esther Rome," in *Boston Women's Health Book Collectives Archives* (Cambridge Mass.: Schlesinger Library on the History of Women, 1995), 2, 3.

32. Boston Women's Health Book Collective, *Menstruation* (Boston: Boston Women's Health Book Collective, 1977), 1, 3.

33. Playtex introduced the deodorant tampon in 1971. Nancy Friedman, *Everything You Must Know about Tampons* (New York: Berkley Books, 1981), 51.

34. Boston Women's Health Book Collective, *Menstruation*, 3.

35. Dan and Lewis, *Menstrual Health in Women's Lives*, 46.

36. Friedman, *Everything You Must Know about Tampons*, 118. That such a rumor persisted even after being soundly discredited attests to the skepticism among women that flourished in the coming years, validated by the industry's neglect and disregard for women's health.

37. Ibid., 118, xiii. I was unable to ascertain the source(s) of the Berkeley Women's Health Collective's information on tampon safety.

38. Parvati, *Hygieia*, 8.

39. Slayton testifies in *Menstruation: Breaking the Silence*, VHS, written and produced by Penny Wheelwright, producer Teresa MacInnes (Starry Night Productions, 1997). I explore cultural feminism in more depth in chapter 4.

40. Tamara Slayton, "About the Author," in *Reclaiming the Menstrual Matrix: Evolving Feminine Wisdom—A Workbook* (Santa Rosa, Calif.: Menstrual Health Foundation, 1990). The claim is inaccurate: As pointed out earlier, Sea Pearls, a small company selling sea sponges as natural tampons, was founded in 1974 and may have been the first alternative menstrual product company in the United States. The website, Tamara Slayton, www.tamaraslayton.com (accessed June 25, 2005), is now defunct. (I am not aware of any connection to the cloth menstrual pad company Glad Rags, founded in 1992.

41. Qtd. in Nancy Reame, "Menstrual Health Products, Practices, and Problems," in *Lifting the Curse of Menstruation*, ed. Golub, 37.

42. This kind of reportage of consumer anxiety combined with the dismissive voice of authority—in this case, unidentified "medical consultants"—continues into the present.

43. Tierno, *The Secret Life of Germs*, 78.

44. Alicia Swasy, *Soap Opera: The Inside Story of Procter & Gamble* (New York: Simon and Schuster, 1993), 133. Interestingly, it was not until the TSS outbreak that large numbers of women concerned about tampon safety began reaching out to feminist health activists, in addition to consumer advocates like Braiman.

45. "General Controls for Medical Devices," http://www.fda.gov/MedicalDevices/DeviceRegulationandGuidance/Overview/GeneralandSpecialControls/ucm055910.htm (accessed June 10, 2009).

46. Meadows, *Tampon Safety*.

47. Tierno, *The Secret Life of Germs*, 75.

48. This product discontinuation marked the company's withdrawal from the tampon business until it bought Tambrands in 1997.

49. Tom Riley, *The Price of a Life: One Woman's Death from Toxic Shock Syndrome* (Bethesda, Md.: Adler and Adler, 1986), 248.

50. Kathleen Shands, G. P. Schmid, and B. B. Dan, "Toxic-Shock Syndrome in Menstruating Women: Association with Tampon Use and Staphylococcus Aureus and Clinical Features in 52 Cases, *New England Journal of Medicine* 25 (1980): 1436–1442.

51. Officials at P&G claim that Tierno's research lacks credibility. Jay Gooch, in interview with the author, Boston, July 22, 2004.

52. Federal Food, Drug, and Cosmetic Act, U.S. Code 21 (1976), § 360.

53. Esther Rome and Jill Wolhandler, "Can Tampon Safety Be Regulated?" in *Menstrual Health in Women's Lives*, ed. Dan and Lewis, 261. *OBOS* advances this opinion in its 1984 edition.

54. Schorr and Conte qtd. in Mayer, *The Consumer Movement*, 49.

55. Boston Women's Book Collective, *Menstruation* (Boston: Boston Women's Health Book Collective, 1981), 2.

56. Boston Women's Health Book Collective, "Letter to Dockets and Management Branch (HPA 305)." In Series X, 56.13–58.2, Correspondence, General, Boston Women's Health Book Collective Archives, Schlesinger Library on the History of Women, Cambridge, Mass. (June 22, 1981).

57. Other consumer groups were recruited and joined the BHWBC. They included Woman Health International and the National Women's Health Network, the Empire State Consumers Association, and the Coalition for the Medical Rights of Women (Rome and Wolhandler, "Can Tampon Safety Be Regulated?" 262).

58. Rome and Wolhandler, "Can Tampon Safety Be Regulated?" 263.

59. Mayer, *The Consumer Movement*, 30.

60. Rome and Wolhandler, "Can Tampon Safety Be Regulated?" 267.

61. Boston Women's Health Book Collective, *Our Bodies, Ourselves: A Book by and for Women* (New York: Simon and Schuster, 1984), 211.

62. Ibid., 211–212.

63. Ibid.

64. Reame, "Menstrual Health Products, Practices, and Problems," 37, 47; "Tamara Slayton," www.tamaraslayton.com (accessed June 25, 2005).

65. Friedman, *Everything You Must Know about Tampons*, 129.

66. "Tampons and Toxic Shock," qtd. in Rome and Wolhandler, "Can Tampon Safety Be Regulated?" 267.

67. Rome and Wolhandler, "Can Tampon Safety Be Regulated?" 267.

68. Qtd. in Lara Owen, *Her Blood Is Gold: Celebrating the Power of Menstruation* (San Francisco: HarperSanFrancisco, 1993), 124.

69. Bernadette Vallely, e-mail interview with the author, November 5, 2003.

70. See Liz Armstrong and Adrienne Scott, *Whitewash: Exposing the Health and Environmental Dangers of Women's Sanitary Products and Disposable Diapers—What You*

Can Do about It! (New York: Harper Perennial, 1992); and Alison Costello, Bernadette Vallely, and Josa Young, *The Sanitary Protection Scandal* (London: Women's Environmental Network, 1989); and Houppert, *The Curse.* In 2004, dioxin's danger was thrust into the public consciousness when Ukrainian presidential candidate (now president) Viktor Yuschenko was found to be a victim of dioxin poisoning resulting in liver, intestinal, and spleen problems and disfiguring facial cysts (Elisabeth Rosenthal, "Liberal Leader from Ukraine Was Poisoned," *New York Times*, December 13, 2004, under "World," http://www.ntimes.com/2004/12/12/international/europe/12ukraine.html?ex= 1120363200anden=1d102c527c2497e5andei=5070 [accessed July 1, 2005]).

71. Vallely interview, November 5, 2003.

72. Ibid.

73. Dowie, *Losing Ground*, xiv.

74. Ibid., 73.

75. Robert Musil, *Hope for a Heated Planet: How Americans Are Fighting Global Warming and Building a Better Future* (New Brunswick, N.J.: Rutgers University Press, 2009), 82, 83.

76. Natracare: History, http://www.natracare.com/p106/en-GB/About-Us/Hisoty.aspx (accessed December 12, 2009).

77. Madeleine Shaw, e-mail interview with the author, April 19, 2006.

78. Cloth Pad Reviews, http://clothpadreviews.makeforum.org/a-z-list-of-all-pads -quick-find-202.html (accessed June 10, 2009).

79. Houppert, *The Curse*, 19.

80. Gooch interview.

81. See www.seac.org/tampons. These data were cited by www.seac.org/tampons before the Tampaction campaign was suspended and web content removed. The campaign is in the process of being revived (Andrew Munn, e-mail to the author, March 9, 2009).

82. Houppert, *The Curse*, 26.

83. Boston Women's Health Book Collective, *The New Our Bodies, Ourselves* (New York: Simon and Schuster, 1992), 250.

84. See Seth F. Berkley, Allen W. Hightower, Claire V. Broome, and Arthur L. Reingold, "The Relationship of Tampon Characteristics to Menstrual Toxic Shock Syndrome," *Journal of the American Medical Association* 258 (1987): 917–920.

85. Even the CDC cites a possible reason for the drop in TSS cases to be "diminished attention to TSS in the medical literature." "Historical Perspectives Reduced Incidence of Menstrual Toxic-Shock Syndrome—United States, 1980–1990," http://www.cdc.gov/ mmwr/preview/mmwrhtml/00001651.htm (accessed June 10, 2009).

86. Jane Wegscheider Hyman and Esther R. Rome, *Sacrificing Our Selves for Love: Why Women Compromise Health and Self-Esteem . . . and How to Stop* (Freedom, Calif.: Crossing Press, 1996).

87. Rome and Wolhandler, "Can Tampon Safety Be Regulated?" 270.

88. Dowie, *Losing Ground*, 261–262.

89. Student Environmental Action Coalition, *We Call for Tampaction!* (Philadelphia: Student Environmental Action Coalition, circa 2005), n.p.

90. Ibid.

4 — FEMINIST-SPIRITUALIST MENSTRUAL ACTIVISM

1. Kami McBride, e-mail interview with the author, July 29, 2005.

2. Anthony Giddens, *Modernity and Self-Identity: Self and Society in the Late Modern Age* (Cambridge: Polity Press, 1991), 214.

3. Jesse J. Helton and William J. Staudenmeier Jr., "Re-imagining Being 'Straight,'" *Contemporary Drug Problems* 29, no. 2 (summer 2002): 463; qtd. in Ross Haenfler, *Straight Edge: HardCore Punk, Clean-Living Youth, and Social Change* (New Brunswick, N.J.: Rutgers University Press, 2006), 79.

4. Living Awareness, http://www.livingawareness.com/ (accessed June 25, 2005). Content no longer available.

5. Carol Christ, *Rebirth of the Goddess: Finding Meaning in Feminist Spirituality* (New York: Routledge, 1997); Starhawk, *The Spiral Dance: A Rebirth of the Ancient Religion of the Great Goddess* (San Francisco: HarperSanFrancisco, 2005); Lucia Chiavola Birnbaum, *She Is Everywhere! An Anthology of Writing in Womanist/Feminist Spirituality* (New York: iUniverse, 2005).

6. Joan Morais, e-mail interview with the author, August 12, 2005. Bernadette Vallely, e-mail interview with the author, November 11, 2005, Vallely's emphasis.

7. Barbara Hannelore, e-mail interview with the author, December 14, 2005.

8. Elayne Doughty, e-mail interview with the author, October 18, 2005.

9. See, for example, Marija Gimbutas, *The Civilization of the Goddess* (San Francisco: Harper and Row, 1991), *The Goddesses and Gods of Old Europe* (San Francisco: Harper and Row, 1974), and *The Language of the Goddess* (San Francisco: Harper and Row, 1989).

10. Hannelore interview.

11. See Red Web Foundation, http://www.redwebfoundation.org.

12. Giddens qtd. in Verta Taylor and Nancy Whittier, "Collective Identity in Social Movement Communities: Lesbian Feminist Mobilization," in *Frontiers in Social Movement Theory*, ed. Aldon Morris and Carol Mueller (New Haven: Yale University Press, 1992), 168.

13. See Hank Johnston, H. Laraña, and Joseph Gusfield, *The New Social Movements* (Philadelphia: Temple University Press, 1994).

14. Haenfler, *Straight Edge*, 62.

15. I offer a more sustained critique of the essentialism central to the feminist-spiritualist wing of the movement in chapter 7.

16. Margaret Bertulli, "I Bleed Therefore I Am" (website now defunct), 2000; reprinted with permission.

17. Owen, *Her Blood Is Gold*, 66.

18. Echols, *Daring to Be Bad*, 264.

19. Ryan, *Feminism and the Women's Movement*, 55; Echols, *Daring to Be Bad*, 244, 243.

20. Echols, *Daring to Be Bad*, 243.

21. Rich, *Of Woman Born*, 11.

22. Red Web Foundation, About Us, http://www.redwebfoundation.org/1.html?SID (accessed June 10, 2009).

23. McBride interview.

24. Chris Bobel, *The Paradox of Natural Mothering* (Philadelphia: Temple University Press, 2002), 164; see also Judith Grant, *Fundamental Feminism: Contesting the Core Concepts of Feminist Theory* (New York: Routledge, 1993), 59–74; Linda Alcoff, "Cultural Feminism versus Post-Structuralism: The Identity Crisis in Feminist Theory," *Signs* 13, no. 3 (Spring 1988): 414.

25. Lorber, *Gender Inequality*, 134

26. The percentages may be even higher. I collected this and other demographic information via a brief questionnaire. In the blank for "your socio-economic status," all but

three of the feminist-spiritualists wrote either "middle class" or "upper middle class." Of the three who did not use this language, one wrote "hmmm," another left the question blank, and the third, a midwife and holistic health educator, referred to herself as "poor in money."

27. Starkweather's conference is a labor of love. She is clear with attendees, in her characteristically honest way, that the conference is a financial hardship for her; the registration fee she charges at best permits her to break even on the event. "The Women's Belly and Womb Conference has not made a profit in years. It is a giant act of service and full of the same resources if not more than those who are 'nonprofits.' Point in case can you imagine that I have done what I've done without grants, tax status, volunteer energy, etc? Just pure will to be a transformative force in these times regardless of whether I will never have a board, endless paperwork and tracking by outside forces as to what I can and cannot do?" E-mail to the author, June 9, 2009.

28. For further information regarding the Belly and Womb Conference: Belly and Womb Conference, http://alisastarkweather.com/index.php?option=com_contentandtask =blogcategoryandid=15andItemid=49. Gender segregation is common to such events. This type of separatism has roots that reach at least into the second wave of the women's movement when lesbian separatists asserted that women-only spaces were necessary to create a context of safety for women, because in mixed-gender settings, sexist dynamics compromise women's agency (for more on lesbian separatism, see Sarah Lucia Hoagland and Julia Penelope, *For Lesbians Only: A Separatist Anthology* (London: Onlywomen, 1988). The most contentious and enduring example of women-only space is, of course, the Michigan Womyn's Music Festival, where I first encountered the Bloodsisters described in the introduction. For an explanation and defense of the policy, see a press release issued by event founder Lisa Vogel, available at http://eminism.org/michigan/ 20060822-mwmf.txt. For information regarding organized protest against this policy, see Camp Trans 2009: Room for All Kinds of Womyn, http://www.camp-trans. org/. I do not engage here the pros and cons of women-only events, but it is important to acknowledge their central place in feminist-spiritual menstrual activism.

29. ALisa Starkweather, "Born from a Woman," *Women Rise Up* (ALisa Starkweather, CD, 2005). Reprinted with permission.

30. Buckley and Gottlieb, *Blood Magic*, 12, 11.

31. Ibid., 12, emphasis in original.

32. The Red Tent, http://theredtent.tribe.net/thread/41dfb9a4–515a-4048-afa4-e6f50d3e489f (accessed June 15, 2009).

33. "Red Tent by Locale," http://alisastarkweather.com/index.php?option=com _content&task=blogcategory&id=29&Itemid=51 (accessed September21, 2009).

34. Sally Price, *Co-Wives and Calabashes* (Ann Arbor: University of Michigan Press, 1984), 113; Sally Price, "The Curse's Blessing," *Frontiers: A Journal of Women Studies* 14, no. 2 (1994): 123–142; quotations on 123, 133.

35. For example, see Ann Crittenden, *The Price of Motherhood: Why the Most Important Job in the World Is Still the Least Valued* (New York: Metropolitan Books, 2001).

36. My reference to Steinem's self-help book is strategic in this context. That even Steinem, the icon of the (white, middle-class) U.S. women's movement, jumped on the self-improvement bandwagon in the early 1990s suggests the nearly magnetic pull of individual-level solutions to systemic problems.

37. Lisa Hogeland, *Feminism and Its Fictions: The Consciousness-Raising Novel and the Women's Liberation Movement* (Philadelphia: University of Pennsylvania Press, 1998), 25.

38. Carol Hanisch, "The Personal Is Political," February 1969, Women and Social Movements in the United States, 1600–2000: The "Second Wave" and Beyond, http://scholar.alexanderstreet.com/pages/viewpage.action?pageId=2259 (accessed June 10, 2009). The Southern Conference Educational Fund (SCEF) hired organizers to explore the viability of establishing a women's liberation project in the South.

39. Shulamith Firestone and Anne Koedt, *Notes from the Second Year Women's Liberation: Major Writings of the Radical Feminists* (New York: Radical Feminism, 1970). Hanisch credits Firestone and Koedt with the title in her memo "The Personal Is Political."

40. ALisa Starkweather, Belly and Womb Conference, conference schedule, Baldwinville, Mass., 2005.

41. Meenakshi Durham, "Displaced Persons: Symbols of South Asian Femininity and the Returned Gaze in U.S. Media Culture," *Communication Theory* 11, no. 2 (2001): 201–217. Mehndi is a form of body decoration popular in south Asia and parts of Africa in which one applies henna, typically to the hands, feet, or both.

42. Sunita Puri, "'Ethnic Fashion' Obscures Cultural Identity," *Yale Herald*, http://www.yaleherald.com/archive/xxxi/2001.02.02/opinion/page12aethnic.html (accessed June 10, 2009).

43. Cultural appropriation occurs when one adopts a cultural practice or theory of a member of another culture as if it were one's own or as if the right of possession should not be questioned or contested, according to Jonathan Hart in "Translating and Resisting Empire: Cultural Appropriation and Postcolonial Studies," in *Borrowed Power: Essays on Cultural Appropriation*, ed. Bruce Ziff and Pratima Rao (New Brunswick, N.J.: Rutgers University Press, 1997), 137–168, 138.

44. Durham, "Displaced Persons," 214, 205.

45. Name withheld, e-mail interview with the author, December 14, 2005.

46. Rosemary Coombe, "The Properties of Culture and the Possession of Identity: Postcolonial Struggle and the Legal Imagination," in *Borrowed Power: Essays on Cultural Appropriations*, ed. Bruce Ziff and Pratima Rao (New Brunswick, N.J.: Rutgers University Press, 1997), 90. A rich literature explores and critiques cultural appropriation; see, for an introduction, Bruce Ziff and Pratima Rao, eds., *Borrowed Power: Essays on Cultural Appropriation* (New Brunswick, N.J.: Rutgers University Press, 1997).

47. Durham, "Displaced Persons," 212.

48. There may be cause for optimism. ALisa Starkweather reports that recently her intensive workshop series "Daughters of the Earth" enrolled 25 women of color among its 142 participants, and portions of program content focused on building a more diverse movement (ALisa Starkweather, e-mail to the author, June 15, 2009).

49. Megan Lalonde, "Menstrual Cycle Charting—A Path to Body Literacy: Basic Principles, Methodologies, and Scientific Underpinnings," lecture, Society for Menstrual Cycle Research Conference, University of British Columbia, Vancouver, B.C., Canada, June 9, 2007.

50. Jerilynn Prior, Yvette Vigna, Susan Barr, Cori Rexworthy, and Brian Lentle, "Cyclic Medroxyprogesterone Treatment Increases Bone Density: A Controlled Trial in Active Women with Menstrual Cycle Disturbances," *American Journal of Medicine* 96 (1994): 521–530. See especially 527–529.

51. Geraldine Matus, "Menstrual Cycle Charting—A Path to Body Literacy: Functions and Applications," lecture, Society for Menstrual Cycle Research Conference, University of British Columbia, Vancouver, B.C., Canada, June 9, 2007.

52. Sheri Winston, phone interview with the author, January 3, 2006.

53. Ibid.

54. Bramwell, "Blood and Milk," 513.

55. Living Awareness, http://www.livingawareness.com/ (accessed June 25, 2005).

56. I draw on Bailey's definition of "privilege": "a particular class of unearned advantages that are systematically created and culturally nourished." Lorraine Code, ed., *Encyclopedia of Feminist Theories* (New York: Routledge, 2000), s.v. "Privilege."

57. Miranda Gray, *Red Moon: Understanding and Using the Gifts of the Menstrual Cycle* (Boston: Element Books, 1994), 2.

58. Kami McBride, 105 Ways to Celebrate Menstruation, (Vacaville, Calif. (P.O. Box 5381, Vacaville 95696): Living Awareness Publications, 2004). . 26, 33

59. The veracity of some claims is questionable. For example and as pointed out earlier, anthropologist Sally Price takes issue with Buckley and Gottlieb's liberal interpretation (in the Introduction to their collection) of the menstrual hut in Suriname she described in her book *Co-wives and Calabashes.*

60. Owen, *Her Blood Is Gold*, 85, 2–3. The book was re-released in 1998 by Crossing Press as *Honoring Menstruation: A Time of Self Renewal.*

61. Alexandra Pope, *The Wild Genie: The Healing Power of Menstruation: A Handbook of Self Care* (Bowral, N.S.W., Australia: Sally Milner, 2001), 19–20, 223–229.

62. Hemitra Crecraft, e-mail to the author, January 24, 2006.

63. Chella Quint, e-mail to the author, June 15, 2009.

64. WomanWisdom, "Back Story," http://www.womanwisdom.com/w_backstory.shtml (accessed June 10, 2009).

65. Celebrate Girls, "New Definition of Womanhood," http://www.celebrategirls.com/womanhood.htm (accessed June 10, 2009)

66. ALisa Starkweather, "A New Woman Walks on the Earth," *Daughter of the Earth* (CD, 1997). Reprinted with permission.

67. Helyanna Brooke and Ann Short, *Instruction Booklet* (San Francisco: Brooke, 1997), 37. Emphasis mine.

68. I thank Gayle Sulik for making this point.

69. Elizabeth Kissling. "Bleeding Out Loud: Communication about Menstruation," *Feminism and Psychology* 6, no. 4:481–504, 499.

70. Alix Olson, *Built Like That* (Mr Lady Records, CD, 2001).

71. Baumgardner and Richards, *Manifesta*, 194.

72. When I attended Women's Wisdom, nineteen women were enrolled in the three-part workshop series. Both Belly and Womb Conferences I attended attracted between sixty and seventy-five women and girls.

73. Elizabeth Kissling, prepublication review of *New Blood*, December 22, 2008.

74. ALisa Starkweather, e-mail to the author, June 9, 2009,
June 15, 2009.

5 — RADICAL MENSTRUATION

1. Yonah EtShalom now identifies as genderqueer and accordingly does not use standard gendered pronouns. During the period narrated here, however, EtShalom identified as a

girl/woman, so I use the pronouns "she" and "her." When I speak of EtShalom since transitioning to genderqueer, I use squir pronouns of choice. Punk, a subculture with roots in punk music, is distinguished by forms of music, ideology, fashion, aesthetics, and lifestyle that resist mainstream culture and champion self-reliance. See Mark Andersen and Mark Jenkins, *Dance of Days: Two Decades of Punk in the Nation's Capital* (New York: Akashic Books, 2001); Lauraine Leblanc, *Pretty in Punk: Girls' Resistance in a Boys' Subculture* (New Brunswick, N.J.: Rutgers University Press, 1999); Craig O'Hara, *The Philosophy of Punk: More than Noise* (London: AK Press, 1999); and Haenfler, *Straight Edge.*

2. Yonah EtShalom, e-mail interview with the author, September 5, 2003.

3. As remarkable as this ignorance may sound coming from someone who volunteered to teach how to make alternative menstrual pads, it reflects the deep distrust of corporations and mainstream practices at the heart of the punk ethic. An attitude of "if it comes from a big national, it must be bad" pervades this subculture.

4. Kristin Garvin, e-mail interview with the author, October 7, 2003. This spelling of "women"—replacing the *e* with a *y*—symbolically detaches (wo)manhood from manhood. My efforts to locate the origins of this spelling failed, but anecdotal evidence points to radical feminists active in the 1970s. Sociologist Mindy Fried, for example, personally remembers that "back in the seventies radical feminists began using this spelling because they didn't want 'men' to be a part of the word describing "'womyn.'" It was representative of a radical break—an emancipation of women of sorts or at least a symbolic separation of "the two genders" (Fried, e-mail to the author, June 21, 2007). Thus, Garvin's use of this spelling in the twenty-first century is yet another signal of continuity across the waves of the women's movement.

5. Courtney Dailey, e-mail interview with the author, August 21, 2003.

6. At this time, Dailey apparently was not aware of the growing environmental justice movement, which moves beyond ecological awareness to address the disproportionate number of environmental burdens shouldered by the culturally disadvantaged. For more information, see, for starters, The Environmental Justice Resource Center at Clark Atlanta University, http://www.ejrc.cau.edu (accessed July 1, 2009).

7. Carol Church, *Whirling Cervix* (e-zine, now defunct), 7.

8. Karen Houppert, "Embarrassed to Death: The Hidden Dangers of the Tampon Industry," *Village Voice*, February 7, 1995, available at S.P.O.T., the Tampon Health website, http://spotsite.org/village.html (accessed June 24, 2009). "Cycle Celebration Crown Kits" refers to Tamara Slayton's home-based line of alternative menstrual products (see chapter 4). I would not include Houppert in the category of radical menstruation activist, although the target of her journalistic exposé was certainly the FemCare industry. Her approach as a journalist is more detached, and her original motivation to explore the FemCare industry, she reports in the article, was stimulated by the rising cost of tampons, not by concern for women's health, the environment, or capitalist exploitation. But since her work is widely cited by activists (in multiple zines, e-zines, websites, and workshops), I include it. An interesting side story illustrates the strength of the menstrual taboo. When Houppert's feature story appeared in the *Village Voice*, the cover carried a photograph of the profile of a woman's torso, a tampon string visibly hanging between her legs. When the issue hit the newsstands, letters of complaint poured in—the most the *Voice* had ever received regarding any single photograph or story it had published (Wheelwright and MacInnes, *Menstruation*, VHS).

9. Walker, introduction, xxxi n57.

10. See http://www.hagrag.com.

11. Marie Abbondanza, *It's Your Fucking Body*, limited-circulation, self-published zine, n.d., 4, 6–7. Note the "womyn" spelling, a parody of second-wave feminist framings of identity. This contrasts, curiously, with radical menstruation activist Kristin Garvin's more sincere use of "womyn" when she expressed the potential of menstrual activism to "empower womyn and change their lives." This discrepancy points to the third-wave feminist ambivalence toward second-wave theory and practice.

12. Emily Biting, in interview with the author, Montreal, August 12, 2006.

13. Leblanc, *Pretty in Punk*, 33. See Leblanc for in-depth descriptions of each punk type. For histories and descriptions of punk, see Andersen and Jenkins, *Dance of Days*; O'Hara, *The Philosophy of Punk*; and Haenfler, *Straight Edge*.

14. Harold Levine and Steven Stumpf, "Statements of Fear through Cultural Symbols: Punk Rock as Reflexive Subculture," *Youth and Society* 14 (June 1983): 417–435, qtd. in Leblanc, *Pretty in Punk*, 63–64.

15. Stephen Duncombe, *Notes from the Underground: Zines and the Politics of Alternative Culture* (London: Verso, 1997), 120.

16. Julia Moskin, "Strict Vegan Ethics, Frosted with Hedonism," *New York Times*, January 27, 2007.

17. Those who identify as "straight edge" (represented as "sXe" or " xXx") pledge to live a clean, "poison-free" life, abstaining from smoking, drinking, and in some cases, caffeine, and sex outside committed relationships. See Haenfler, *Straight Edge*.

18. Leo qtd. in Moskin, "Strict Vegan Ethics."

19. From The Bloodsisters Project, www.bloodsisters.org/bloodsisters (accessed May 24, 2004). Reprinted with permission. "Guerrilla girl" is likely a reference to the activist group the Guerilla Girls, who anonymously (their identities are obscured by gorilla masks) call out the underrepresentation of women and people of color in the art world. When I interviewed Bloodsister Emily Biting in Montreal on August 12, 2006, she indicated that there was discussion of changing the group's name to eliminate the word "sister." Sadly, the Bloodsisters disbanded in early 2007.

20. Brackin "Firecracker" Camp, e-mail to the author, August 26, 2003.

21. Dailey interview.

22. Rep. Maloney Introduces Bill to Protect Women from Toxic Shock Syndrome, http://maloney.house.gov/index.php?option=com_content&task=view&id=1564&Itemid =61 (accessed September 9, 2009),

23. The figures cited here are based on a 2006 Nonwovens Industry Report, "Sanitary Protection in the U.S.," http://www.nonwovens-industry.com/articles/2006/11/sanitary -protection-in-the-us (accessed June 24, 2009).

24. Global Industry Analysts, Inc., "Feminine Hygiene Products—Global Strategic Business Report (April 2008)." The term "emerging markets" here refers to rapidly expanding capitalist economies in countries such as Brazil, Russia, India, and China. This usage may originate in Jeffrey E. Garten's *The Big 10: Big Emerging Markets and How They Will Change Our Lives* (New York: Basic Books, 1997).

25. "Sanitary Protection in the U.S." In spite of industry decline (due only to a shifting demographic), most women are held captive to FemCare's products. Each time I talk about my work, women express surprise that alternatives to single-use pads and tampons exist. Typically, after I introduce an audience to the array of options menstrual activists promote, several people make such remarks as: "I never knew any of this. How could I not know this stuff?"

26. Based on 2002 data (the latest available from each of the four U.S.-based companies), Procter & Gamble holds 37 percent of the market share; Kimberly-Clark, 23 percent; Johnson & Johnson, 18 percent; Playtex, 12 percent; and "others," the remaining 10 percent. Eileen Wubbe, "Feminine Hygiene Market Update," Nonwovens Industry (November 2001), www.nonwovens-industry.com/articles/2002/11/feminine-hygiene -market-update.php (accessed July 12, 2007).

27. See Welcome to Tampax, http://www.tampax.com/home.php, and "Our Products .Pads: Ultra Thin Super with Wings," http://www.kotexfits.com/ourProducts/pads/ ultraThinSuperWithWings/.

28. Playtex 2006 Annual Report, 4, http://ww3.ics.adp.com/streetlink_data/dirPYX/ annual/HTML1/default.htm; Jill Rivkin, "Finding the Feminine Approach," *Private Label Buyer*, August 2005, 32.

29. Rivkin, "Finding the Feminine Approach," 30, 32.

30. Eileen Wubbe, "Hygiene Marketing Report," http://www.nonwovens-industry. com/articles/2002/11/feminine-hygiene-market-update (accessed September 16, 2009).

31. "Sanitary Protection in the U.S."

32. From www.seac.org/tampons/ (accessed July 12, 2004). Website no longer available.

33. Tampons and Asbestos, Dioxin, & Toxic Shock Syndrome, http://www.fda.gov/ MedicalDevices/Safety/AlertsandNotices/PatientAlerts/ucm070003.htm (accessed June 15, 2009).

34. L. A. Kauffman, "The Anti-Politics of Identity," *Socialist Review* 90 (1990): 78; Biting interview.

35. Deb (pseudonym), e-mail interview with the author, October 28, 2003; interview with the author, Montreal, August 12, 2006.

36. Reger, *Different Wavelengths*, xxi.

37. Hogeland, *Feminism and Its Fictions*, 10.

38. Duncombe, *Notes from the Underground*, 6–7.

39. V. Vale, ed., *Zines!* Vol. 1 (San Francisco: V Search, n.d.), 4 (emphases in original).

40. Dawn Bates and Maureen McHugh, "Zines: Voices of Third Wave Feminists," in *Different Wavelengths*, ed. Reger, 180; Margaret J. Finders, "Queens, Teen Zines and Early Adolescence: Females Realizing Their Way toward Adulthood," *Anthropology and Education Quarterly* 27, no. 96:71–89, qtd. in ibid., 185.
Susan Lurie, Ann Cvetkovich, Jane Gallop, Tania Modleski, and Hortense Spillers, "Roundtable: Restoring Feminist Politics to Poststructuralist Critique," *Feminist Studies* 27, no. 3 (2001): 702.

41. Duncombe, *Notes from the Underground*, 36, 28, 29.

42. For example, see Vale, *Zines!*.

43. Julie Chu, "Navigating the Media Environment: How Youth Claim a Place through Zines," *Social Justice* 24, no. 3 (1997), 71–85.

44. Bates and McHugh, "Zines," in *Different Wavelengths*, ed. Reger.

45. Reger, *Different Wavelengths*, xxii.

46. Women's Media Transformed by Internet, http://www.womensenews.org/ article.cfm?aid=1201.

47. Echols, *Daring to Be Bad*, 139–158.

48. "Redstockings Manifesto," reprinted in Wendy Kolmar and Frances Bartkowski, eds., *Feminist Theory: A Reader* (London: Routledge, 1969), 179 Cutting Remarks, http:// www.thenation.com/doc/20040614/dederer (accessed June 24, 2009).

49. Qualities of a bitch include: "aggressive, assertive, domineering, overbearing, strong-minded, spiteful, hostile, direct, blunt, candid, obnoxious, thick-skinned, hard-headed, vicious, dogmatic, competent, competitive, pushy, loud-mouthed, independent, stubborn, demanding, manipulative, egoistic, driven, achieving, overwhelming, threatening, scary, ambitious, tough, brassy, masculine, boisterous, and turbulent." "The Bitch Manifesto," http://www.jofreeman.com/joreen/bitch.htm (accessed September 21, 2009).

50. S.P.O.T. stands for Stop Poisoning Our Twats, language Bannett feared would turn away some visitors to her Web page and so refrained from spelling out (Tracy Bannett, phone interview with the author, July 15, 2003). Curiously, Bannett mistitles Houppert's article "Embarrassed to Death" as "Pulling the Plug on the Sanitary Protection Industry"). See "Pulling the Plug on the Sanitary Protection Industry," http://www.spotsite.org/.

51. Federation, *A New View*, 123.

52. Houppert, "Embarrassed to Death."

53. Naomi Klein, *No Logo: Taking Aim at the Brand Bullies* (New York: Picador, 1999), 280. The term "culture jamming" was coined in 1984 by the San Francisco–based band Negativland.

54. Kalle Lasn, *Culture Jam: The Uncooling of America* (New York: Eagle Brook, 1999). Lasn is the founder of *Adbusters* magazine, a periodical devoted to challenging consumerism through culture jamming.

55. Friedman qtd. in Vince Carducci, "'Culture Jamming': A Sociological Perspective," *Journal of Consumer Culture* 6, no. 1 (2006): 132.

56. Adventures in Menstruating, www.chartyourcycle.co.uk (accessed April 21, 2009).

57. Margaret Farrar and Jamie Warner, "Rah-Rah-Radical: The Radical Cheerleaders' Challenge to the Public Sphere," *Politics and Gender* 2 (2006): 281.

58. "Sparkle Motion!" http://radcheer.uproot.info (accessed June 15, 2009).

59. Brackin "Firecracker" Camp and StikiNiki "Blood Cheer" (1999), in *Femmenstruation Rites Rag: Stories of Wimmin's Blood and Rites of Passage*, (self-published zine, n.d., 19. Reprinted with permission. Camp and collaborators Cara Jennings, Jeanne Vaccaro, and Karolina Bång are at work on an anthology on radical cheerleading. See http://www.rararadical.com.

60. Ladyfest is a not-for-profit festival of music and arts intended to showcase the talent of women and girls. Rooted in the underground scene, the first Ladyfest took place in Olympia, Washington, in 2000. Since then Ladyfests have occurred all over the world, especially in the United States and Europe.

61. Echols, *Daring to Be Bad*, 94. As students of women's history know, no bras were burned during this protest; however, burning the contents of the Freedom Trash Can was planned until Atlantic City officials banned the action, considered a hazard to the wooden boardwalks beneath the feet of the demonstrators.

62. Jo Freeman, "No More Miss America! (1968–1969)," http://uic.edu/orgs/cwluher story/jofreeman/photos/MissAm1969.html (accessed September 21, 2009).

63. Echols, *Daring to Be Bad*, 389.

64. Jo Freeman, "W.I.T.C.H.—The Womens International Terrorist Conspiracy from Hell," http://www.jofreeman.com/photos/witch.html (accessed June 15, 2009).

65. Ibid.

66. Kristin Garvin, e-mail interview with the author, October 17, 2003.

67. The source for this fanciful list of menstrual cycle euphemisms is now defunct. It was http:// www.chicklit.com/words/words1.html.

68. Also countering this perception are feminist comics such as Kate Clinton, Elvira Kurt, Margaret Cho, and Karen Williams, and the comedic art activism of the Guerrilla Girls.

69. "Menstrual Monday 2009," *http://www.moltx.org/mmindex*1.html (accessed September 22, 2009). Kachman does not identify herself explicitly as an activist (much less a "radical menstruation" activist) or her work as activism, and Strange self-identifies as a "feminist filmmaker mom" whose focus is female centered. But because their work refuses mainstream framings of menstruation and promotes a menstruation-positive view that urges women to embrace, rather than reject, their embodiment, I include Menstrual Monday as an example of radical menstruation activism.

70. Using single-use products to raise awareness about their evils may seem a curious choice, given the radical menstruation push to boycott such products. Because this contradiction was not apparent to me at the time of my fieldwork, I did not ask the activists to explain their choice. But I suspect they would argue that the number of tampons used to make one crown hardly compares to the number of tampons the typical menstruator would use if s/he had not been alerted to their hazards.

71. Liz Armstrong, e-mail interview with the author, November 11, 2003.

72. Jay Critchley, e-mail communication with the author, September 22, 2009.

73. Siobhán O'Connor, "Pussy Power: Bloodsisters Marks Its Fourth Anniversary with Permanent New Digs in Mile-End," *Montreal Mirror, The Front,* March 2, 2000 (accessed April 18, 2009). Is selling gear activism? Some have their doubts, as I discussed in chapter 4. Emily Biting, a member of the Bloodsisters Collective, shared a story with me in our August 12, 2006, interview that brought out this tension. While Biting was selling Urban Amour products at an anarchist book fair, a woman chided her: "You are selling panties. That's not activism." Here, it is not clear if the fact of selling anything was challenged or the selling of panties, in particular. However, the Bloodsisters are explicit that the sale of their products supports their activism. And I would add that *someone* must sell menstrual product alternatives if the call to seek out substitutes to conventional products is to bear any weight. Might it be better still if the entity selling them is a small not-for-profit DIY feminist collective?

74. Gloria Kaufman, introduction to *Pulling Our Own Strings: Feminist Humor and Satire,* ed. Gloria Kaufman and Mary Kay Blakely (Bloomington: Indiana University Press, 1980). 16.

75. Gloria Steinem, "If Men Could Menstruate," in *Pulling Our Own Strings,* ed. Gloria Kaufman and Mary Kay Blakely (Bloomington: Indiana University Press, 1980), 25–26.

76. I resist lumping the feminist-spiritualist and radical menstruation workshops together because of one significant difference: The feminist-spiritualist workshops engage participants in ideological change, modeling and urging the adoption of an alternative, positive (and essentialist) view of menstruation that holds the potential for self-transformation, while the radical menstruation workshops promote conceptual change *and* add an action-based component that not only benefits individual menstruators, but also supports the environment and resists corporate control.

77. It is noteworthy that tampon applicators are typically not included in European tampon products. In Japan, however, Elldy introduced finger cots in the 1990s. According to Museum of Menstruation curator Harry Finley, the cots enable women to insert their tampons without making direct contact with their vaginas. See "Japanese menstrual tampon with finger cots (Elldy tampons), 1990," http://www.mum.org/japfgrtn.htm (accessed July 1, 2009).

78. As I (ineptly) stitched together my own pad, I was reminded of the sewing societies of the nineteenth century, where, according to feminist legend, women surreptitiously hatched strategies for gaining suffrage and staged other gender-based social change actions. Today, a popular t-shirt worn by young feminists reads "Ladies Sewing Circle and Terrorist Society." The same text appears on the back cover of one of the Bloodsisters' zines.

79. Zimmerman, "The Women's Health Movement," 442–472, 455.

80. See Judy Norsigian, Viluynya Diskin, Paula Doress-Wortens, Jane Pincus, Wendy Sanford, and Norma Swenson, "The Boston Women's Health Book Collective and Our Bodies, Ourselves: A Brief History and Reflection," *Journal of the American Women's Medical Association* 54 (1999): 35–39; Laura Kaplan, *The Story of Jane: The Legendary Underground Feminist Abortion Service* (New York: Pantheon Books, 1995); and Federation, *A New View.*

81. adee took issue with this analysis. When I shared the penultimate draft of this book with her, she wrote me a lengthy letter admitting that she was "sensitive to some of [my] (open-ended) conclusions—that the radical side of menstrual activism does not contextualize the spectrum of the work we inherited in terms of feminist/environmentalism and social activism—from the past." She went on to list the myriad influences for the founding of the project, including feminist art, the fields of gender studies and political science, and antiglobalization and antimultinational politics. She notes: "We made a conscious effort to attend to those complexities of such matters as second and first wave feminisms . . . sometimes endorsed by humour . . . or referring to the issues of americanized feminisms of the past with analysis and respect and put in perspective in framing currents [*sic*] field of activisms" (e-mail to the author, June 9, 2009).

6 — MAKING SENSE OF MOVEMENT PARTICIPATION

1. Baumgarder and Richards, *Manifesta*, 283.

2. Since completing my research on natural mothering, I have identified a more diverse population of natural mothers, including lesbian mothers, single mothers, poor mothers, and mothers of color. It is possible that the natural-mothering population has always been more diverse that I initially discovered, but due to my own social location and my raced, classed, and otherwise particularized framing of natural mothering, I did not see the movement fully. It is also possible the movement has grown and changed (even mainstreamed, as I argue elsewhere—see Chris Bobel, "Resisting, But Not Too Much: Interrogating the Paradox of Mothering," in *Maternal Theory: Essential Readings 1976–2007*, ed. Andrea O'Reilly (Toronto: Demeter Press, 2007), 782–791, making it more appealing and more accessible to a wider cross-section of mothers. It remains, however, a lifestyle most readily accessible to those with privilege.

3. Cultural capital refers to the amassing of resources, such as forms of knowledge, skills, attitudes, and education, that are societal recognized and valued and thus confer power and status; see Pierre Bourdieu, "The Forms of Capital," in *Handbook of Theory and Research for the Sociology of Education*, ed. J. G. Richardson (New York: Greenwood. Press, 1986), 241–258.

4. Carol Church, e-mail interview with the author, January 23, 2006.

5. See appendix C. The precise number of college attendees is not included in the table because the data for this measure were unreliable. Curiously, ten of the sixty-five respondents did not answer this question. Based on anecdotal evidence collected in the field and

revealed during interviews, however, I am confident in describing the studied population as overwhelmingly college educated.

6. In certain progressive contexts such as social justice organizations, it might be said that self-identifying as queer is itself a political choice and one that more accurately reflects an ideological than a sexual orientation. That is, for some activists—especially those exposed to burgeoning queer theory and energized by gender activism, which, generally speaking, seeks to undo gender as we know it—claiming themselves queer signals a political stance in support of expression unbounded by gender and sexualities. As some feminists claimed a lesbian identity for political reasons (although they were not sexually attracted to women and lived as straight women) during the second wave (e.g., see Dorothy Allison, "Conceptual Lesbian," in *Surface Tension: Love, Sex, and Politics between Lesbian and Straight Women* [New York: Simon and Schuster, 1996], 147), today feminists and other progressives may claim the disparaged identity of "queer." The limits of this study do not permit me to explore this possibility, however. I thank Jyoti Puri for suggesting this line of inquiry. See appendix C for demographic information on the sixty-five interview participants.

7. Why does this activist, committed to menstrual health and politics, not regard resisting unsafe femcare and supporting health and wellness a matter of "basic survival"? I thank Amie "Breeze" Harper for raising this question.

8. Sarah (pseudonym), e-mail interview with the author, July 6, 2005.

9. I reluctantly use the overly broad term "women of color" to refer to women in the United States who identify as African American or Black, Asian American, indigenous or Native American, Latina, biracial, or multiracial. While using the global term "women of color" constructs a false monolith by erasing the divergent histories and life experiences of women from each of these subcategories, I use it here because it remains the standard English-language term to refer to women who are not white and/or Euro-American.

10. Rosabeth Moss Kanter, *Men and Women of the Corporation* (New York: Basic Books, 1977), 63; Leblanc, *Pretty in Punk*, 64.

11. Lynn Roberts, Loretta Ross, and M. Bahati Kuumba, "The Reproductive Health and Sexual Rights of Women of Color: Still Building a Movement," *NWSA Journal* 17, no. 1 (2005): 94.

12. On reproductive justice, for example, see Jael Silliman, Marlene Gerber Fried, Loretta Ross, and Elena Gutiérrez, *Undivided Rights: Women of Color Organize for Reproductive Justice* (Cambridge, Mass.: South End Press, 2004); and Jennifer Nelson, *Women of Color and the Reproductive Rights Movement* (New York: New York University Press, 2003). On AIDS, see, for example, Cathy Cohen, "Punks, Bulldaggers, and Welfare Queens," *Gay Lesbian Quarterly* 3 (1997): 437–465; and Brett Stockdill, *Activism against AIDS: At the Intersections of Sexuality, Race, Gender, and Class* (Boulder, Colo.: Lynne Reiner, 2003)

13. Patricia McKeever, "The Perpetuation of Menstrual Shame: Implications and Directions," *Women and Health* 9, no. 5 (1984): 33–47; Dorothy Hawthorne, "Symbols of Menarche Identified by African American Females," *Western Journal of Nursing Research* 24, no. 5 (2002): 486; Shirley Dashiff, "Education for Menarche," *Journal of School Health* 56, no. 2 (1986): 56–60, 67; Elisha Nixon, Phyllis Kenoff Mansfield, Linda A. Kittell, and Sandra L. Faulkner, "'Staying Strong': How Low-Income Rural African American Women Manage Their Menopausal Changes," *Women and Health* 34, no. 2 (2001): 84.

14. Clarissa Scott, "The Relationship between Beliefs about the Menstrual Cycle and Choice of Fertility Regulating Methods within Five Ethnic Groups," *International Journal of Gynaecology and Obstetrics* 13 (1975): 105–109; Nancy Woods, Gretchen Dery, and Ada Most, "Recollections of Menarche, Current Menstrual Attitudes, and Perimenstrual Symptoms," in *Menarche*, ed. Sharon Golub (Lexington, Mass.: Lexington Books, 1983), 87–98; and Janet Lee and Jennifer Sasse-Coen, *Blood Stories: Menarche and the Politics of the Female Body in Contemporary U.S. Society* (New York: Routledge, 2006), 44.

15. Women of Color Web, http://www.hsph.harvard.edu/grhf/WoC/ (accessed May 25, 2007).

16. More recently, a search on the Asian-Pacific Resource and Research Centre for Women website produced two hits referencing the health hazards associate with the menstrual taboo in South Asia: http://arrow.org.my/home (accessed December 14, 2009).

17. The URLs for the websites are http://www.gurl.com, http://www.plannedparenthood .org/teen-talk/, and http://www.youngwomenshealth.org.

18. Arnold Farr, "6 Whiteness Visible," in *What White Looks Like: African American Philosophers on the Whiteness Question*, ed. George Yancy (New York: Routledge, 2004), 144; Amie "Breeze" Harper, e-mail interview with the author, July 29, 2007.

19. Harper interview.

20. Helynna Brooke, e-mail interview with the author, August 26, 2005.

21. Amie "Breeze" Harper hypothesizes that my failure to locate larger numbers of menstrual activists of color rested in part with my use of the term "menstrual activism," which may not resonate for many women. She posted queries (using the language "holistic womb health") to several health-oriented Black cybercommunities. Within a few hours of posting, she wrote me the following e-mail (February 15, 2007): "So far, 4 women have written me back about holistic womb health. I think that's the key phrase. When I initially wrote 'menstrual activism' in the subject head, months ago, that was not 'appealing' to the women in this group. However, the phrase holistic womb health is a much more accessible term and the women on the 5 Black-oriented whole foods vegan sites instantly know what I'm referring to."

22. I thank Kevin Allred for making this point.

23. Sharon Powell, e-mail interview with the author, May 31, 2007.

24. For more information about the ethical travesty of the Tuskegee Syphilis Study, see Susan Reverby, *Tuskegee's Truths: Rethinking the Tuskegee Syphilis Study* (Chapel Hill: University of North Carolina Press, 2000).

25. Nixon et al., "'Staying Strong,'" 89.

26. Higginbotham, *Righteous Discontent*, 196.

27. Ibid., 204.

28. Dorothy Roberts, *Killing the Black Body: Race, Reproduction and the Meaning of Liberation* (New York: Pantheon, 1997), 4; Patricia Hill Collins, *Black Sexual Politics: African Americans, Gender and the New Racism* (New York: Routledge, 2004), 138–139, 177, 178.

29. Hawthorne, "Symbols of Menarche," 493.

30. The study used for comparison was Diane Ruble and Jeanne Brooks-Gunn's "The Experience of Menarche," *Child Development* 53, No. 6, Early Adolescence (December 1982): 1557–1566. Scott et al. used the same measurement in their study of Black girls. See Clarissa Scott, D. Arthur, R. Owen, and M. I. Panizo, "Black Adolescents' Emotional Response to Menarche," *Journal of the National Medical Association* 81, no. 3 (1989): 285–290.

31. Scott, "The Relationship between Beliefs," 288.

32. Hawthorne, "Symbols of Menarche," 487–488. This dropout rate is especially remarkable given that each mother-daughter pair was selected based on a "willingness and ability to communicate in focused conversation about menarche."

33. M. L. Poland and G. E. Beane, "A Study of the Effects of Folklore about the Body on IUD Use by Black American Adolescents," *Contraceptive Delivery Systems* 1, no. 4 (October 1980): 333–340, qtd. in Scott, "The Relationship between Beliefs," 289.

34. Interview with Amie "Breeze" Harper, July 29, 2007, emphases in original.

35. Opeyemi Parham, e-mail interview with the author, May 12, 2007. Lisa Fishbayn, a fellow visiting research associate at the Women's Studies Research Center at Brandeis University, alerted me to the Zimbabwean "Dignity. Period!" campaign, which may provide another illustration of the social mandate to uphold respectability through "appropriate" menstrual care. One effect of the severe economic crisis in Zimbabwe has been the soaring costs of FemCare products, now priced out of reach for most women. Many Zimbabwean women can no longer afford single-use products. Instead, they are forced to use cotton wool, newspapers, and dirty rags to manage their monthly menses, options that the women find repellant and a risk to their health (ACTSA: Action for South Africa, http://www.actsa.org/page-1022-Dignity!%20Period.html [accessed July 1, 2009]). In 2005 Action for Southern Africa (ACTSA) in collaboration with the Zimbabwe Congress of Trade Unions initiated a campaign, "Dignity! Period," to deliver disposable FemCare products to women in need. From a North American menstrual activist perspective, shipping tons of donated environmentally unfriendly, unhealthy FemCare products to Zimbabwe is an unfortunate and short-sighted solution to the problem. The amount of waste left behind by these single-use products is staggering, and the potential hazards associated with conventional products are concerning. But from a Zimbabwean perspective, there are no other viable options. With precious clean water in short supply, alternative FemCare such as cloth pads, cups, and sponges are simply unrealistic. I doubt that Zimbabwean women would use alternative FemCare even if they could, because there is much more at stake in this campaign. Women's lack of access to proper female products puts their very respectability in question. If women cannot manage their menstruation discreetly, in line with the modern standard practices they've grown accustomed to, their very dignity, as the campaign name demonstrates, is compromised. As a "Dignity! Period" campaign leaflet states: "Women have to choose between feeding their families and keeping their dignity." Again, in order to maintain the status of respectable, the menstruating body must be controlled and concealed. For women who are forced to struggle *as* women (given the economic crisis that is a daily feature of Zimbabwean life), the mess of menstruation must be contained and concealed.

36. Matt Reitman, e-mail interview with the author, June 30, 2005.

37. Michael Warner, *Fear of a Queer Planet: Queer Politics and Social Theory* (Minneapolis: University of Minnesota Press, 1993), xiii, emphases mine; Gamson, "Must Identity Movements Self-Destruct?" 250; Warner, *Fear of a Queer Planet*, xxvii.

38. Winston interview.

39. Rachel Warner, e-mail interview with the author, August 5, 2005 Gamson, "Must Identity Movements Self-Destruct?" 253.

40. Chella Quint, e-mail interview with the author, May 17, 2009. Proposition 8 was a California ballot measure that changed the state constitution to read: "Only marriage between a woman and a man is valid or recognized in California." It passed in November 2008 and dealt a major blow to queer marriage campaigns everywhere.

41. Cohen, "Punks," 447. In this piece, Cohen asserts that the label "queer" is "fraught with unspoken assumptions which inhibit the radical potential of this category." In her interactions with LGBT people of color, she has found that "queer" is read as a term rooted in class, race, and gender privilege and thus articulates a politics based on narrow sexual dichotomies that make no room either for the analysis of oppression of those we might categorize as heterosexual or for the privilege of those who operate as queer (451).

7 — WHEN "WOMEN" BECOMES "MENSTRUATORS"

1. I am indebted to MinJeong Kim, who graciously translated the Korean voiceover into English.

2. In parts of East Asia, particularly Japan and Korea, inoffensive terms for those who exist outside the rigid two-gender/two-sex system have recently entered the lexicon. For example, *futanari* (meaning "two form" and usually referring to intersexuals) and *newhalf* (usually referring to a pre-op transwoman) are considered polite terms. Both originate from the Japanese anime and manga world of stylized character types. Harisu is often referred to as a newhalf, or sometimes as a shemale, the latter considered a vulgar term. The source for this information is not reliable, however; see "Futanari," http://en.wikipedia.org/wiki/Futanari (accessed July 1, 2009).

3. Su-cheol Hwang, "Transgender Singer to Do Menstrual Pad Ads," *Chosun Ilbo*, http://english.chosun.com/data////.htm (accessed April 14, 2004).

4. What is less clear to me in this commercial is the meaning of the cryptic voiceover: "There is something that I really want to do . . ." What is this something? Does Harisu speak as a transsexual, perhaps as someone who wishes for a biological woman's body that could menstruate and bear children? Or is she speaking as a woman in the general sense, a woman who wants to fall in love or be sexually (or otherwise) adventurous. This ambiguity is intriguing. For another, more recent gender play on menstruation, see Tampax's viral video series (complete with blog and a Twitter account) *Zack at 16*, in which a teen boy wakes up to discover he has "girl parts" and in a matter of days experiences his first menstruation. The campaign is an ingenious platform for stealth marketing of Tampax products, particularly in the "Help Me" section of the website, where contributors offer advice to Zack regarding menstrual product use. Notably, Tampax Pearl is mentioned repeatedly as posters' product of choice. See http:// www.zack16.com.

5. Johanna Foster, "An Invitation to Dialogue: Clarifying the Position of Feminist Gender Theory in Relation to Sexual Difference Theory," *Gender and Society* 13, no. 4 (1999): 431–456, 450.

6. Ibid., 444.

7. I am not suggesting that only radical menstruation activists apply gender theory in their activism. Certainly, transgender and intersex rights activists, such as those active in GenderPac and the Intersex Society of North America (to name only two major organizations), have been doing this work for years. What I find uniquely important about radical menstruation is the way it queers gender vis-à-vis a *biological process* that is, culturally speaking, practically synonymous with womanhood. If menstruation can be queered, given the strength of its gendered and sexed associations, this may suggest a new frontier. Joining gender-bending pioneers such as Leslie Feinberg, Riki Wilchins, Cheryl Chase, and Kate Bornstein, and numerous activists who follow in their footsteps, the radical menstruation activists destabilize the veracity of gender as rooted in and defined by the biological body.

8. Alcoff, "Cultural Feminism," 405–436, 435.

9. Here, I am using Judith Lorber's definitions of sex and gender. Sex refers to the bio-logical or, more precisely, "the complex interplay of genes, hormones, environment and behavior. Gender refers to a social status, a legal designation, and a personal sense of iden-tity" (Lorber, *Gender Inequality*, 9).

10. Esther Rome and Jill Wolhandler, "Letter to Women," *Boston Women's Health Book Collective Archives* (Cambridge, Mass.: Schlesinger Library on the History of Women, 1985).

11. Of course, there is not a single transcommunity but many transcommunities shaped by intersecting identities. I use the term here to reference a general, loosely allied network of transidentified and transpositive allies who share some common language, including the term "biowoman," which refers to a person born with standard primary and second-ary sex characteristics designated female. In *Whipping Girl: A Transsexual Woman on Sexism and the Scapegoating of Femininity* (Seattle: Seal Press, 2007), Julia Serano coins antonyms, using "cisgender" synomously with "nontransgender" and "cissexual" with "nontranssexual" (33).

12. "Transgender Korean Singer to Market Menstrual Pads," Summer 2004, http://Transgenderonline.com/.html (accessed July 11, 2007).

13. P. Fawn, *Red Scare*, no. 3, self-published zine, 2001, n.p.

"M to F" (like "M2F" and "MtF") is shorthand for "male-to-female transgendered per-son"; "F to M," "F2M," and "FtM" connote a male-to-female transgendered person. I use the abbreviations MtF and FtM in my own writing. I use the word "trans" throughout this chapter as defined by transrights activist Emi Koyama in "The Transfeminist Manifesto": "'Trans' is often referred to as an inclusive term encompassing a wide range of gender norm violations that involve some discontinuity between the sex a person is assigned at birth and her or his gender identity and expression" (244).

14. Abbondanza, *It's Your Fucking Body*, no. 2, n.d. Through the course of this work, I've found the "not only women menstruate and not all women menstruate" statement a puzzle to many people, confirming the embedded relationship of womanhood and men-struation. To clarify, some transmen still menstruate (even on masculinizing hormone treatments, amenorrhea is not immediate and breakthrough bleeding does sometimes occur). Some transmen do not wish to eliminate their periods, often for health reasons. See, for instance, *Period: The End of Menstruation* (DVD, directed and produced by Giovanna Chesler, La Jolla, Calif.: G6 Pictures, 2006), a documentary on the menstrual suppression debate, which narrates the story of Morty Diamond, a transman who titrates his testosterone intake to preserve his capacity to menstruate. Postoperative transwomen who have vaginas (and take feminizing hormones) lack uteri; thus they do not menstru-ate. Some intersexuals who identify as women may lack either uteri or vaginas (and thus do not menstruate), while some intersexuals who identify as men may possess the biolog-ical capacity to menstruate.

15. "Student Environmental Action Coalition (SEAC)," Tampaction, http://www .seac.org/ (accessed October 31, 2004).

16. Yonah EtShalom, Below the Belt Center for Sexual, Genital, and Reproductive Health, http://www.deadletters.biz//.html#who (accessed July 21, 2005). Website now defunct. A slightly revised version of this statement (also authored by EtShalom) appears in the SEAC campaign's Tampaction packet (Student Environmental Action Coalition, *Tampaction Packet* [Philadelphia: Student Environmental Action Coalition, 2003]). The

alternative spelling of "women" (similar in spirit to "womyn") used throughout EtShalom's document reflects again, I would argue, third-wave feminism's tenuous relationship with second-wave feminism. At the same time EtShalom endeavors to disconnect menstruation from the gendered body (a third-wave project), squee deploys language that distinguishes women from men—a practice begun during the development of radical feminism of the 1970s.

17. This push for transinclusion also presents an opportunity to engage extant discussions about what some would call sexism in some corners of the FtM movement. The wholesale rejection of their femininity is profound for some transmen. See, for example, Jason Cromwell, *Transmen and FTMSs: Identities, Bodies, Genders, and Sexualities* (Urbana: University of Illinois Press, 1999); Holly Devor, *FTM: Female-to-Male Transsexuals in Society* (Bloomington: Indiana University Press, 1997); Judith Halberstam, *Female Masculinity* (Durham, N.C.: Duke University Press, 1998); and Henry Rubin, *Self-Made Men: Identity and Embodiment among Transsexual Men* (Nashville: Vanderbilt University Press, 2003). While I did not find an antifemininity sentiment motivating (mostly nontrans-led) menstrual activism, it is important to be alert to this possibility. I thank Doreen Drury for making this point.

18. An activist from Wisconsin told me she was working on a pattern for cloth menstrual pads designed to fit inside boxer shorts because she wanted the transmen she knew to have access to sustainable and safe menstrual care.

19. Devor, *FTM*, 195. Devor now identifies as a transman, Aaron Devor, but because the source I cite is published under the name Holly Devor, I use that name and the appropriate pronouns.

20. Rubin, *Self-Made Men*, 110.

21. Source withheld; emphases in original. To protect the anonymity of the person I quote here, I do not name her website, nor do I name the websites that host the open-access discussion boards I studied.

22. In this context, "passing" refers to the ability of a transperson to succeed at being read by others as belonging to her or his chosen gender. That is, a transman passes if others—particularly strangers—see him as a man.

23. Leong, "Living outside the Box," 101.

24. Susan Stryker, "Transgender Feminism: Queering the Woman Question," in Gillis, Howie, and Munford, *Third Wave Feminism*, 63, 64. I hope not to imply that transgender issues serve only (or primarily) as a vehicle through which theorists can make more sophisticated claims or activists can organize more effectively; transgender theorizing must focus on the ultimate goal of improving the quality of transgendered lives. My aim is to make clear how third-wave feminism's attention to transinclusion has both practical and conceptual implications.

25. Judith Butler, *Undoing Gender* (New York: Routledge, 2004), 212.

26. Judith Butler, *Gender Trouble: Feminism and the Subversion of Identity* (New York: Routledge, 1990), 11.

27. Peter Osborne and Lynne Segal, "Gender as Performance: An Interview with Judith Butler," London, 1993, extracts at http://www.theory.org.uk/but-int1.htm, n.p. Full version originally published in *Radical Philosophy* 67 (summer 1994): 32–33.

28. Butler, *Gender Trouble*, viii.

29. Rosi Braidotti, *Nomadic Subjects: Embodiment and Sexual Difference in Feminist Theory* (New York: Columbia University Press, 1994), 169. Braidotti in particular rejects

the characterization of sexual difference theory as fundamentally essentialist. In fact, early in *Nomadic Subjects*, she clarifies that sexual difference theory construes embodiment "as neither a biological or a sociological category but rather as a point of overlapping between the physical, the symbolic, and the sociological." That is, she claims, sexual difference theory is not biologically determinist, but it does uphold female subjectivity as indispensable and fundamental and the point from which women can and should resist oppression. This is precisely the position the feminist-spiritualist menstrual activists take.

30. My gratitude is owed to Christine Cooper, who coined the phrase "living Butler" during one of our many discussions about this book in progress.

31. Ransom qtd. in Rachel Alsop, Annette Fitzsimmons, and Kathleen Lennon, *Theorizing Gender* (Malden, Mass.: Polity Press, 2002), 221.

32. See Alcoff, "Cultural Feminism," 405–436; Braidotti, *Nomadic Subjects*; Butler, *Bodies That Matter*; Diana Fuss, *Essentially Speaking: Feminism, Nature, and Difference* (New York: Routledge, 1989); Barbara Ryan, ed., *Identity Politics in the Women's Movement* (New York: New York University Press, 2001); Schor and Weed, *The Essential Difference*.

33. Alsop et al., *Theorizing Gender*, 221.

34. Gamson, "Must Identity Movements Self-Destruct? " 249, 259, emphasis in original.

35. Diana Fuss, *Essentially Speaking: Feminism, Nature, and Difference* (New York: Routledge, 1989); Butler, *Undoing Gender*, 192.

36. adee (The Bloodsisters Project), "We Are," 1996; reprinted in *Femmenstruation Rites Rag: Stories of Wimmin's Blood and Rites of Passage*, self-published zine, n.d., 38. Reprinted with permission. Given the context, I interpret "goddess thumpers" as a play on "Bible thumpers." I do not interpret it to describe those who assault (even metaphorically) Goddess worshippers. The reference to "feminist terrorist" is pre-9/11 and was intended to parody the stereotype of the so-called scary feminist (adee, e-mail to the author, May 16, 2009).

37. adee, e-mail to the author, June 15, 2009.

CONCLUSION

1. Kinser, "Negotiating Spaces for/through Third-Wave Feminism," 128–29.

2. Leila Rupp and Verta Taylor, *Survival in the Doldrums: The American Women's Movement* (Princeton, N.J.: Princeton University Press, 1987).

3. Baumgardner and Richards, *Manifesta*, 17.

4. Troy Duster, "'Buried Alive': The Concept of Race in Science," in *Intersections of Gender, Race, and Class: Readings for a Changing Landscape*, ed. Marcia Texler Segal and Theresa A. Martinez (Los Angeles: Roxbury, 2007), 498, 500.

5. Elsewhere, I challenge the assumption that collective action necessarily depends on alignment between personal identity and collective identity. Some social movement participants, including many of those I dubbed menstrual activists, resist the identity "activist" yet find themselves caught "being activist" and "doing activism." See Chris Bobel, " 'I'm Not an Activist, Though I've Done a Lot of It': Doing Activism, Being Activist, and the 'Perfect Standard' in a Contemporary Movement," *Social Movement Studies* 6:2 (2007): 147–159.

6. Lily, e-mail interview with the author, January 1, 2004.

7. An even more recent advertising campaign for cycle-stopping contraception makes clear the contrast between those who try menstrual suppression and those holding out. On the home page of www.periodslessoften.ca (the work of an anonymous "research-based

pharmaceutical company"), a teeny purple thong hangs alongside a pair of extra-large beige briefs on a clothesline.

8. CBS News, "Birth Control with a Boost: A Pill Up for FDA Approval Would Put a Stop to a Woman's Menstruation," http://www.cbsnews.com/stories/2007/05/21/eveningnews/main2833285.shtml (accessed June 11, 2009).

9. See, for example, Johnston-Robledo, Barnack, and Wares, "Kiss Your Period Good-Bye."

10. Rita Arditti and Tatiana Schreiber, "Breast Cancer: The Environmental Connection— A 1998 Update," in *Women's Lives: Multicultural Perspectives*, ed. Gwyn Kirk and Margo Okazawa-Rey, 2nd ed. (Mountain View, Calif.: Mayfield, 2001), 378.

11. Powell interview.

APPENDIX A. METHODS

1. Trying on the role of menstrual activist, I later gave such a workshop based on what I had learned about menstrual health and alternative femcare from the activists I studied. More than thirty students showed up and stitched their own reusable cloth pads (a large turnout on our commuter campus).

2. "Tampaction: Mission Statement," www.seac.org/tampons/misson_statement (accessed June 24, 2004).

3. As pointed out earlier, the majority of the interviewees are white. They are also largely female, college-educated, and under forty and claim a variety of class backgrounds. Nearly half identify as lesbian, gay, or bisexual, most preferring the label "queer." See appendix C for the full demographic profile of those interviewed.

4. See Anselm Strauss and Juliet Corbin, *Basics of Qualitative Research: Techniques and Procedures for Developing Grounded Theory* (Newbury Park, Calif.: Sage, 1998). I acknowledge the irony of my research methods here, in particular the act of creating new categories while pointing out the instability and lack of utility of some extant ones.

5. Ibid., 6.

Index

Page numbers in *italics* refer to figures.

National Women's Political Caucus, 50
National Women's Studies Association Journal, 17, 139
Native American: traditions, xiii, 73–74, 79–80, 81, 90; women, 138, 139, 143. *See also* women of color
Native American Women's Health Education Resource Center, 139, 140
Natracare, 59
natural mothers, 135–136, 216n2
naval gazing, 19
negativity as mandate of menstruation, 31–31
New Age movement, 84–86
New Cycle Products, 52, 102
New England Free Press, 44
New England Journal of Medicine, 53
newhalf, 220n2
New Moon Rising: Reclaiming the Sacred Rites of Menstruation (Wind), 87
The New Our Bodies, Ourselves (BWHBC), 61–62
new racism, 146
new social movements, 66, 69
New York Times, 7, 39–40, 43
New Zealand, 60
NIH. *See* National Institutes of Health
Niki, Stiki, 122–123
Nixon, Elisha, 139, 144
Nixon, Richard, 124
Noble, Vicki, 65, 68
NO LOGO (Klein), 119
Nomadic Subjects: Embodiment and Sexual Difference in Feminist Theory (Braidotti), 166
No More Periods? The Risks of Menstrual Suppression and Other Cutting-Edge Issues about Hormones and Women's Health (Rako), 201n47
Norsigian, Judy, 55
nose rings, 78
Notes from the Second Year (Firestone and Koedt), 77, 117
Not My Mother's Sister: Generational Conflict and Third-Wave Feminism (Henry), 15, 17
NOW. *See* National Organization for Women
NWHN. *See* National Women's Health Network
NWSA Journal, 17, 139

OB (tampon), 107
Obama, Barak, 200n31
Of Co-Wives and Calabashes (Price), 75

Of Woman Born (Rich), 72
O'Hara, Craig, 104
Ohio Women's Rights Convention (1851), 18
Olivia Records, 172
Olson, Alix, 92–93
Olympia Press, 116
Once a Month: Understanding and Treating PMS (Dalton and Holton), 36
105 Ways to Celebrate Menstruation (McBride), 86
Orr, Catherine, 4, 19, 24–25
osteoporosis, 40, 201n47, 202n50
Our Bodies, Ourselves (BWHBC), 41, 42, 44, 47–48, 50–53, 55–56, 62, 117
Owen, Lara, 70, 72–73, 87
Owner's Manual: The Personal, the Political (EtShalom), 98

pads. *See* menstrual pads
Pads4Girls, 59
P&G. *See* Procter & Gamble
Paperwork Reduction Act, 61
The Paradox of Natural Mothering (Bobel), 135
Parham, Opeyemi, 78, 82, 140, 147
participatory research, 185
Parvati Baker, Jeannine, 51–52, 65, 172
passing, transgender term, 164, 222n22
Pearl (tampon), 108
pelvic infections, 49
period extraction, 43, 48, 50, 52, 117
Period Piece (short film), 48, 203n21
Period. The End of Menstruation? (Chesler), 40, 67
"The Personal Is Political," 77
personalized politics. *See* self-help care
personal transformation. *See* self-help care
PersuAsian (periodical), 157
pesticides, 45, 63
Philadelphia Women's Spirituality, 89
Philosophy of Punk: More than Noise! (O'Hara), 104
Piepmeier, Alison, 16, 17, 25
the Pill. *See* hormonal contraception/birth control
Pissed Off Women (POW), 150
Planned Parenthood, 140
plastic surgery, 39
Playtex, 57, 107
Plexus (newspaper), 116
PMDD. *See* Premenstrual Dysphoric Disorder

About the Author

CHRIS BOBEL is an associate professor and the chair of women's studies at University of Massachusetts Boston. Bobel's research engages the intersection of feminist politics, everyday activism, and the body. The author of *The Paradox of Natural Mothering*, Bobel is currently at work on an edited collection (with Samantha Kwan) that explores the body as a site of resistance. She lives with her two daughters and partner outside Boston.